HUMAN ANATOMY
Coloring Book

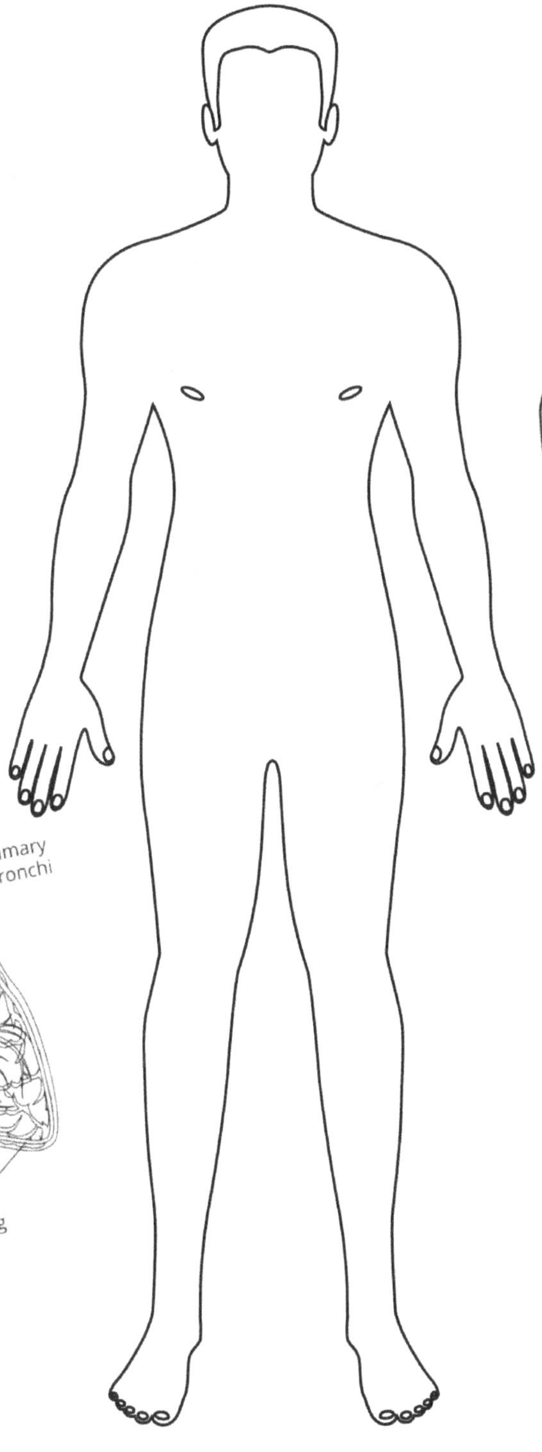

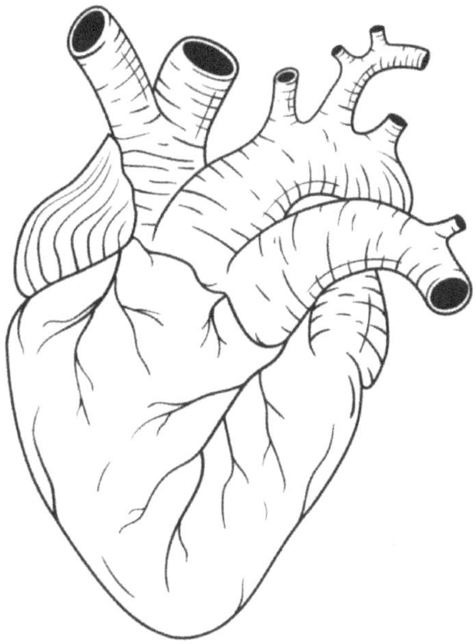

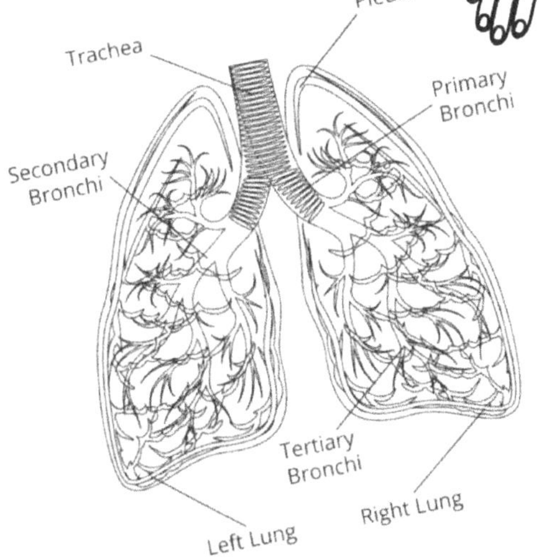

Trachea

Pleura

Primary Bronchi

Secondary Bronchi

Tertiary Bronchi

Left Lung

Right Lung

THE EASIEST WAY TO LEARN HUMAN
ANATOMY.
YOU HAVE THE FREEDOM TO LEARN
THE ANATOMY IN
A FUN AND MEMORABLE WAY.

ISBN: 9798866560622

TABLE OF CONTENTS

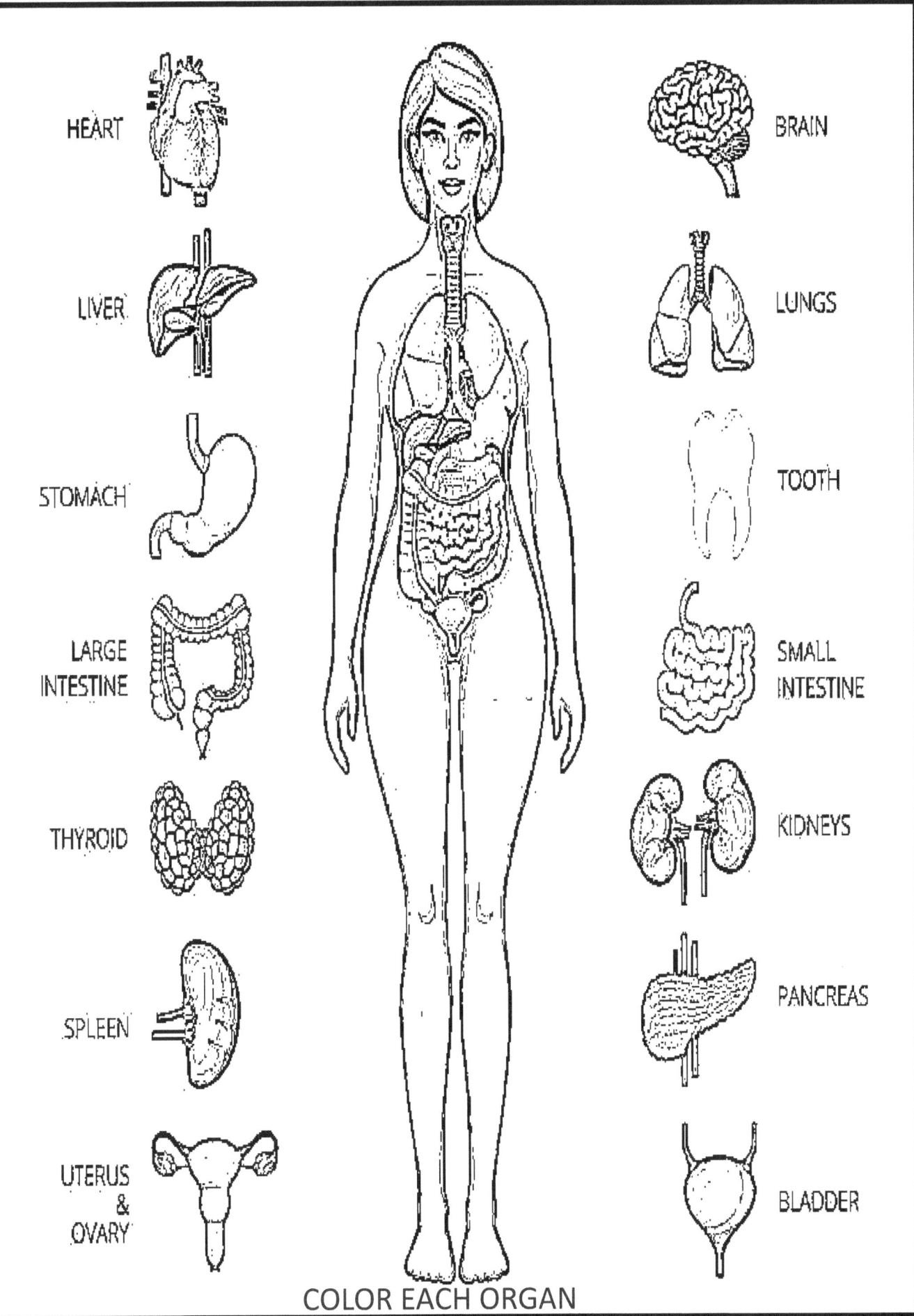

HEART

LIVER

STOMACH

LARGE
INTESTINE

THYROID

SPLEEN

UTERUS
&
OVARY

BRAIN

LUNGS

TOOTH

SMALL
INTESTINE

KIDNEYS

PANCREAS

BLADDER

COLOR EACH ORGAN

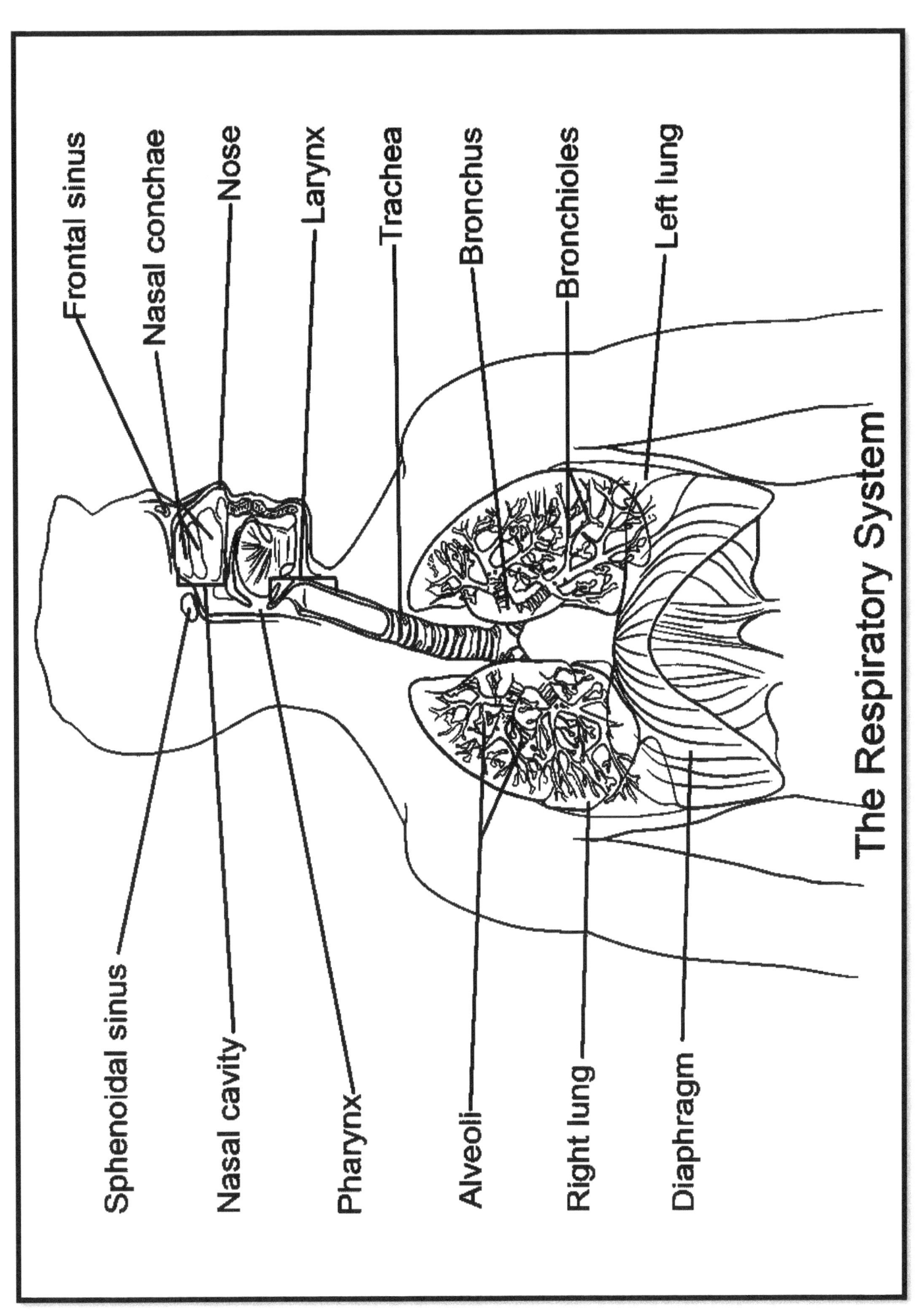

Frontal sinus

Nasal conchae

Nose

Larynx

Trachea

Bronchus

Bronchioles

Left lung

Sphenoidal sinus

Nasal cavity

Pharynx

Alveoli

Right lung

Diaphragm

The Respiratory System

FEMAL VAGINA SYSTEM

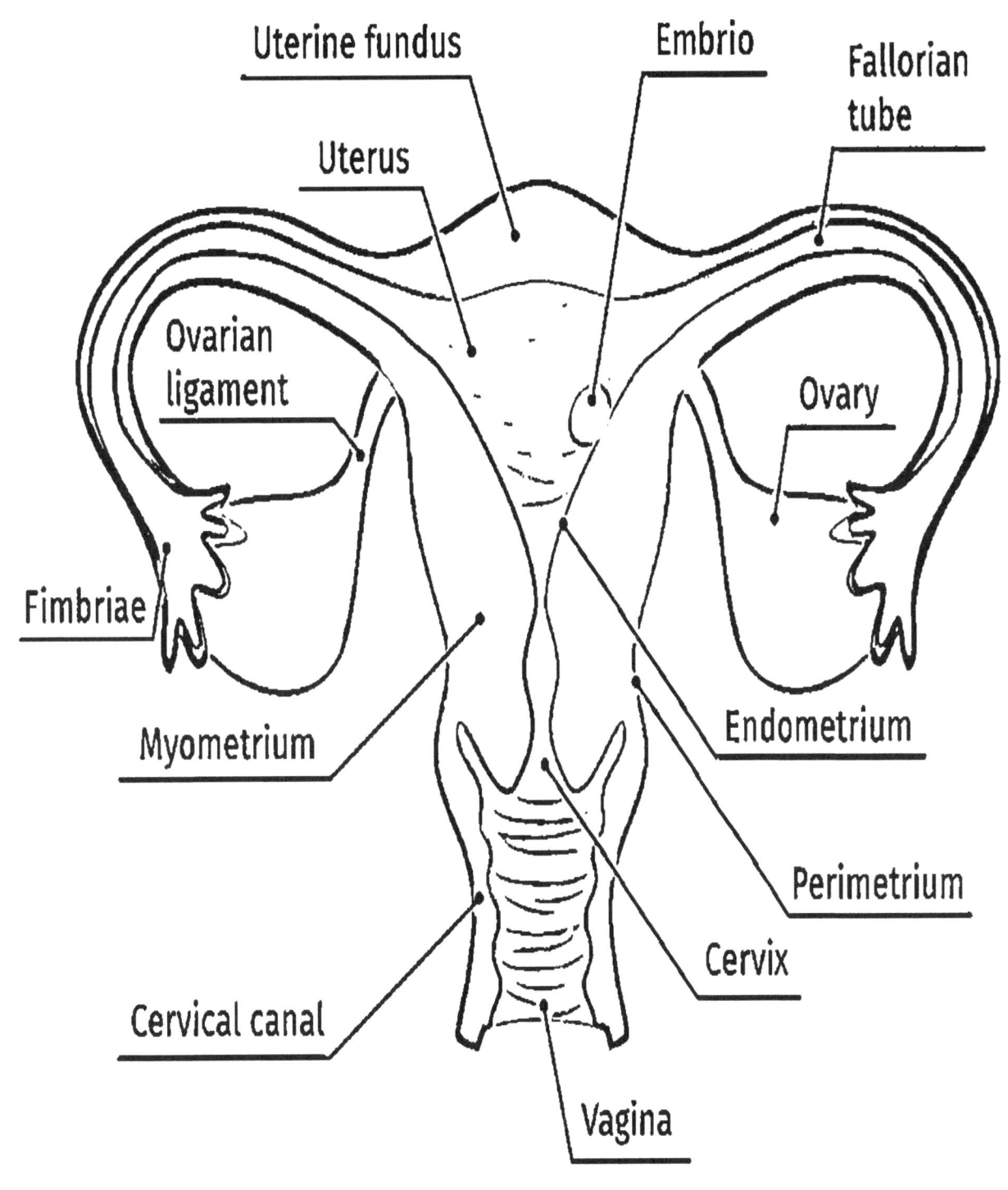

Uterine fundus

Embrio

Fallorian tube

Uterus

Ovarian ligament

Ovary

Fimbriae

Myometrium

Endometrium

Perimetrium

Cervix

Cervical canal

Vagina

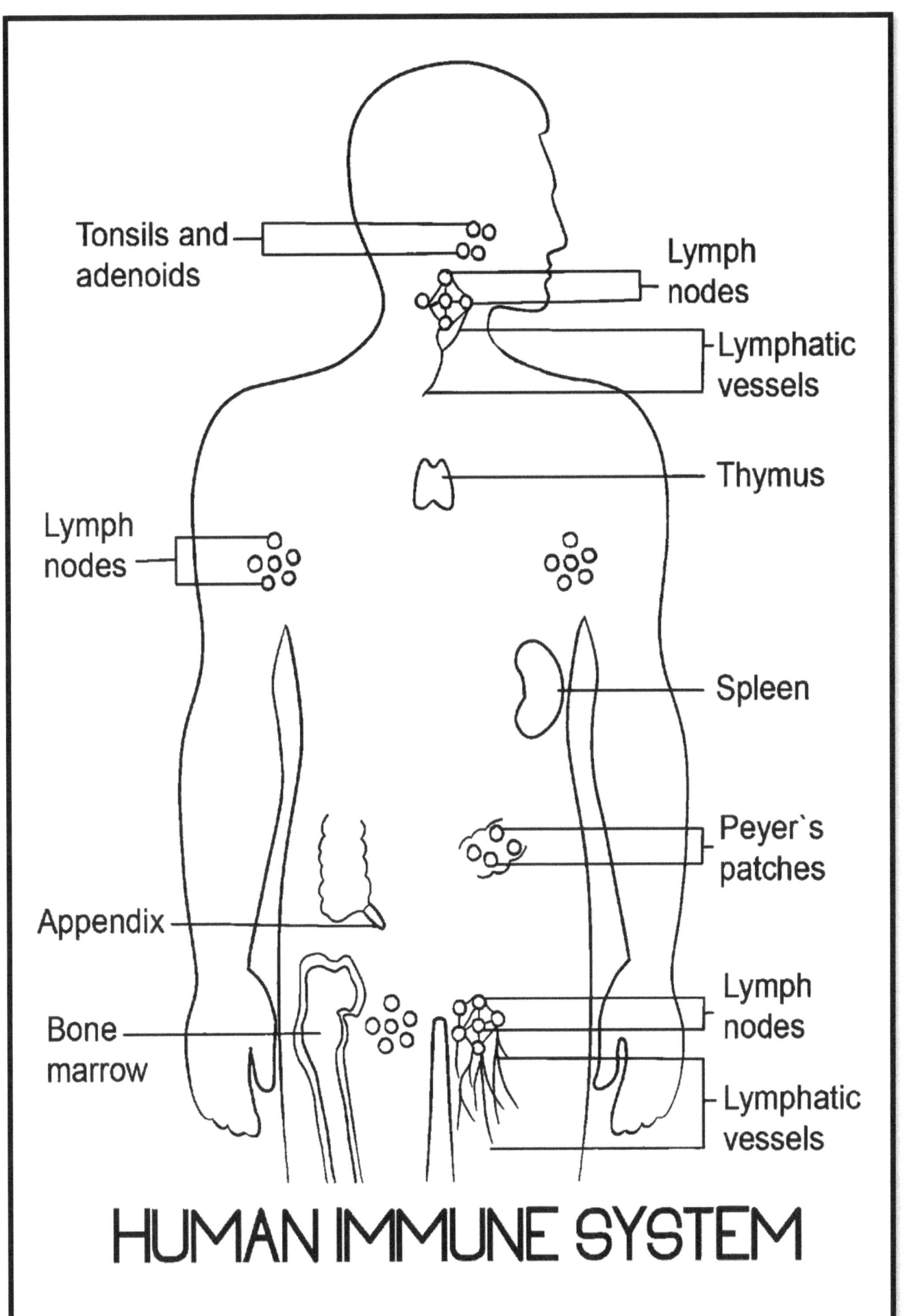

Tonsils and adenoids

Lymph nodes

Lymphatic vessels

Thymus

Lymph nodes

Spleen

Peyer`s patches

Appendix

Lymph nodes

Bone marrow

Lymphatic vessels

HUMAN IMMUNE SYSTEM

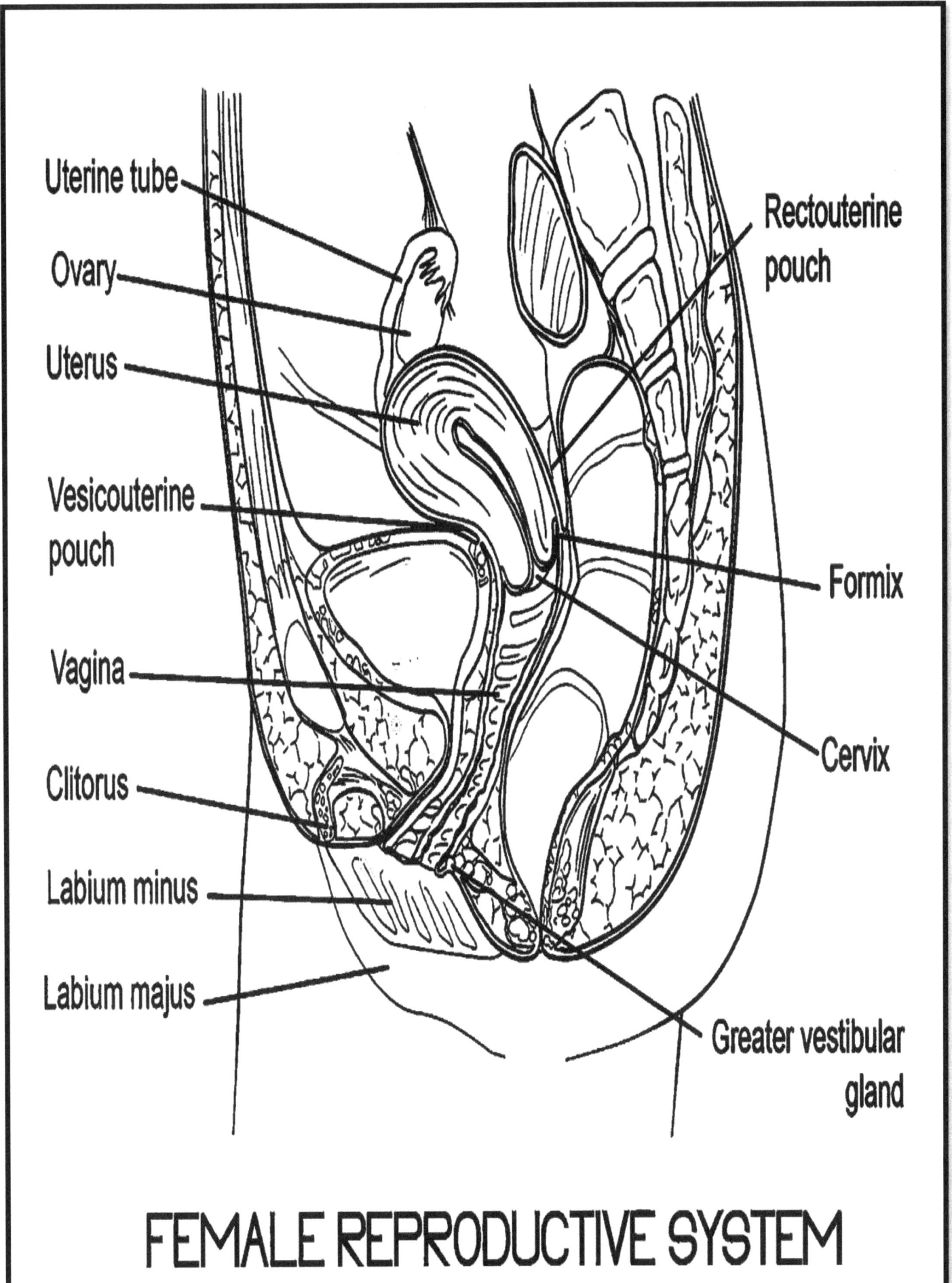

Uterine tube

Ovary

Uterus

Vesicouterine
pouch

Vagina

Clitorus

Labium minus

Labium majus

Rectouterine
pouch

Formix

Cervix

Greater vestibular
gland

FEMALE REPRODUCTIVE SYSTEM

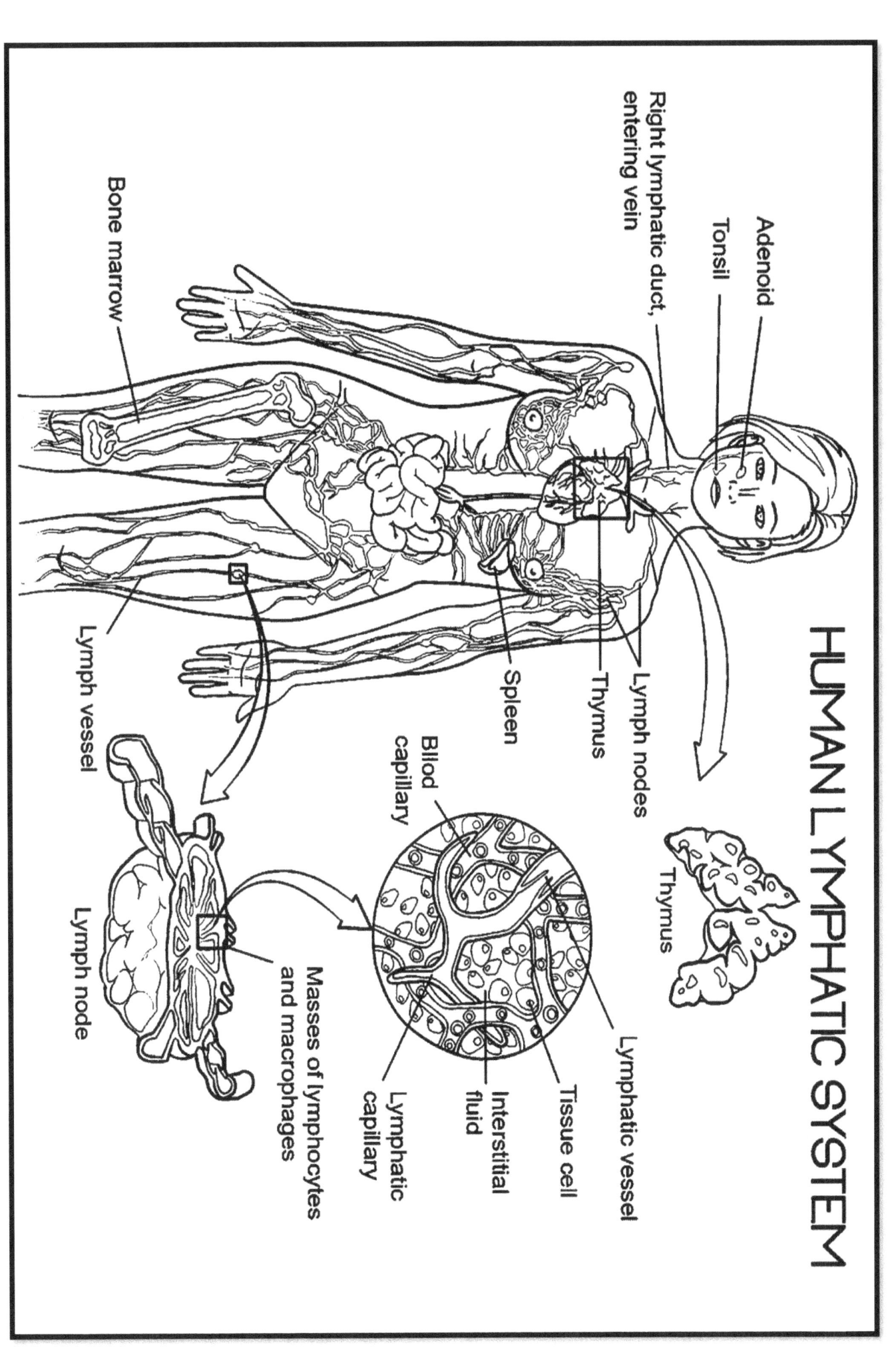

HUMAN LYMPHATIC SYSTEM

Adenoid

Tonsil

Right llymphatic duct, entering vein

Bone marrow

Thymus

Lymph nodes

Thymus

Spleen

Lymphatic vessel

Lymph vessel

Lymph node

Bllod capillary

Masses of lymphocytes and macrophages

Lymphatic capillary

Interstitial fluid

Tissue cell

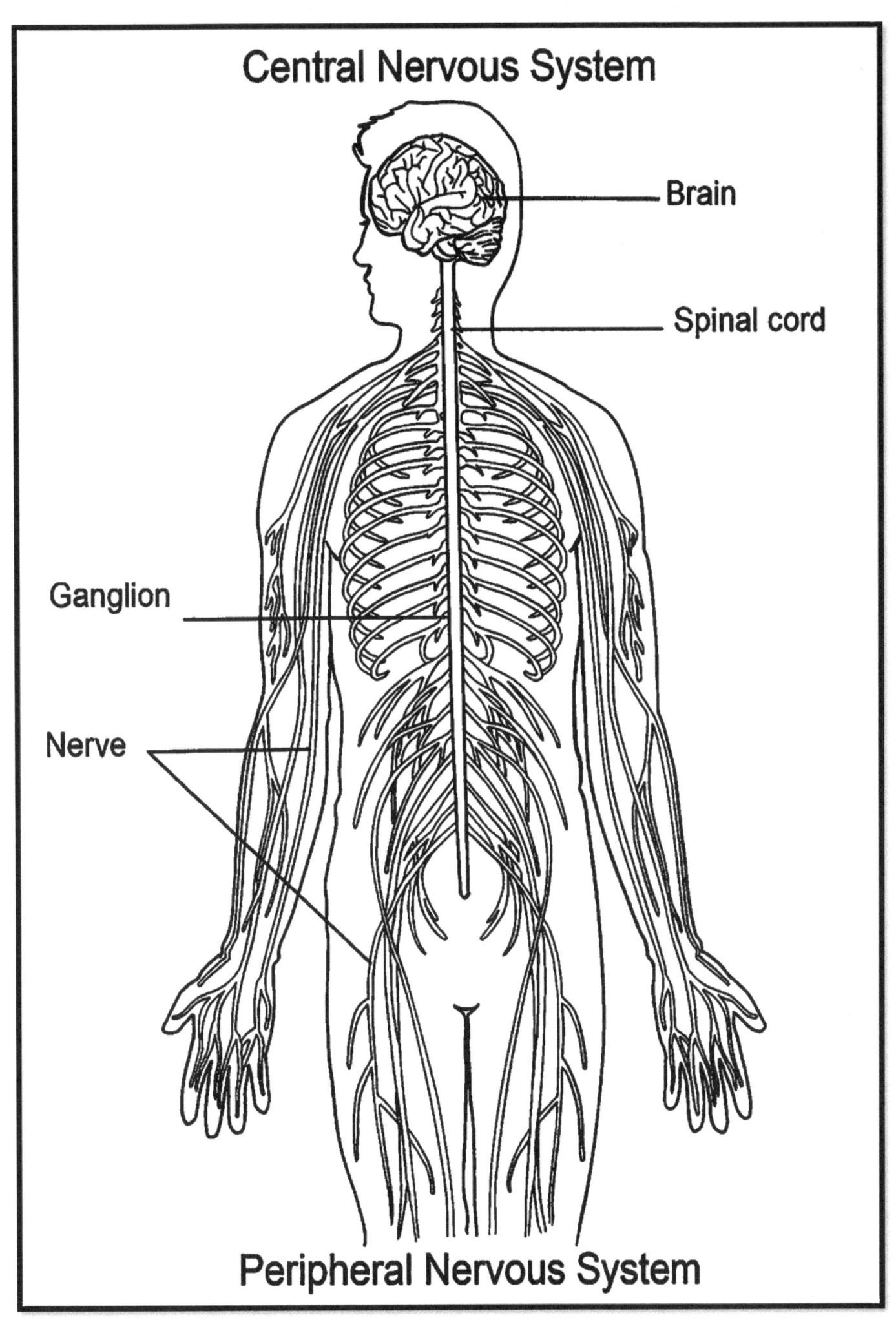

SKELETAL SYSTEM

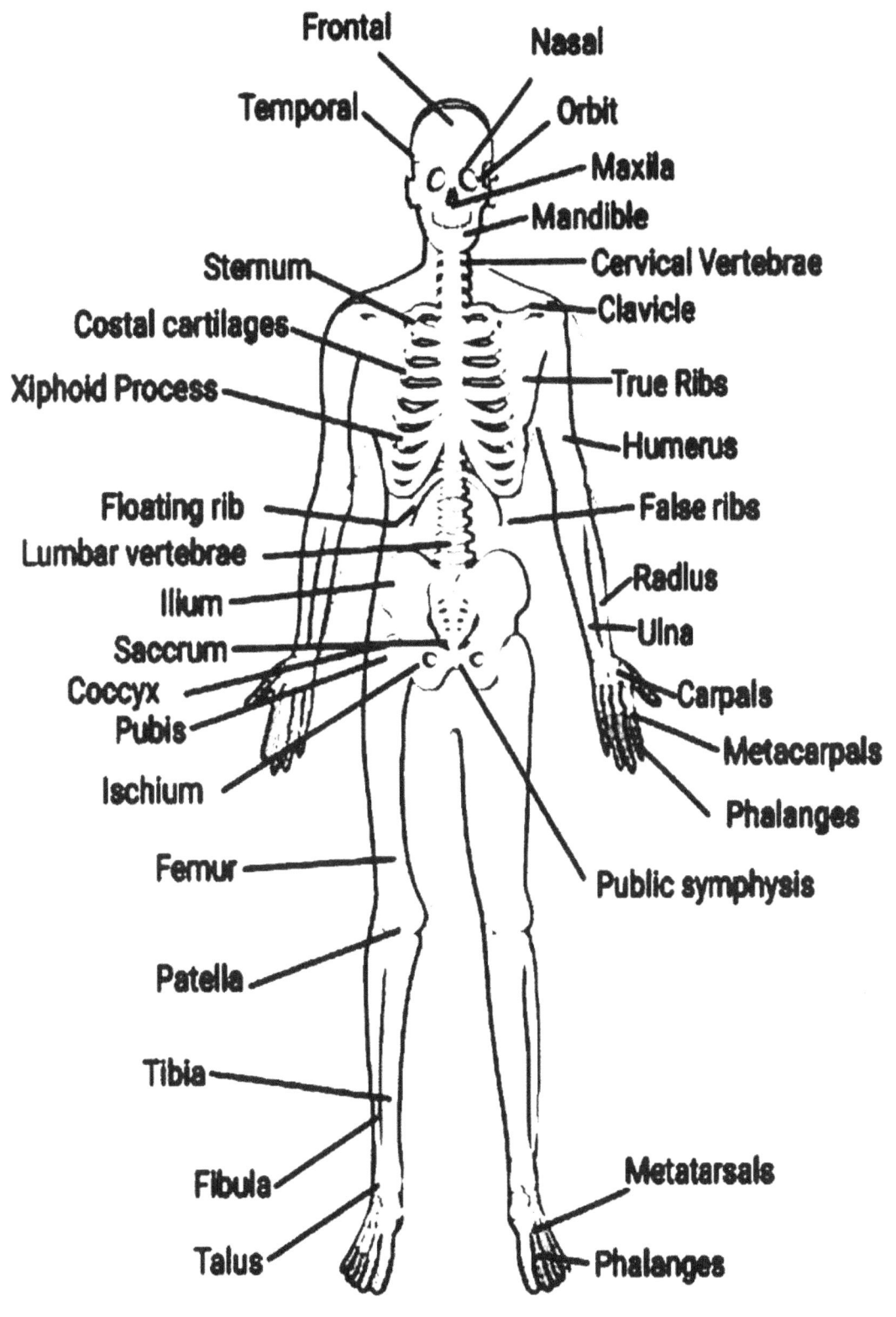

Frontal
Nasal
Temporal
Orbit
Maxila
Mandible
Sternum
Cervical Vertebrae
Costal cartilages
Clavicle
Xiphoid Process
True Ribs
Humerus
Floating rib
False ribs
Lumbar vertebrae
Radlus
Ilium
Ulna
Saccrum
Coccyx
Carpals
Pubis
Metacarpals
Ischium
Phalanges
Femur
Public symphysis
Patella
Tibia
Fibula
Metatarsals
Talus
Phalanges

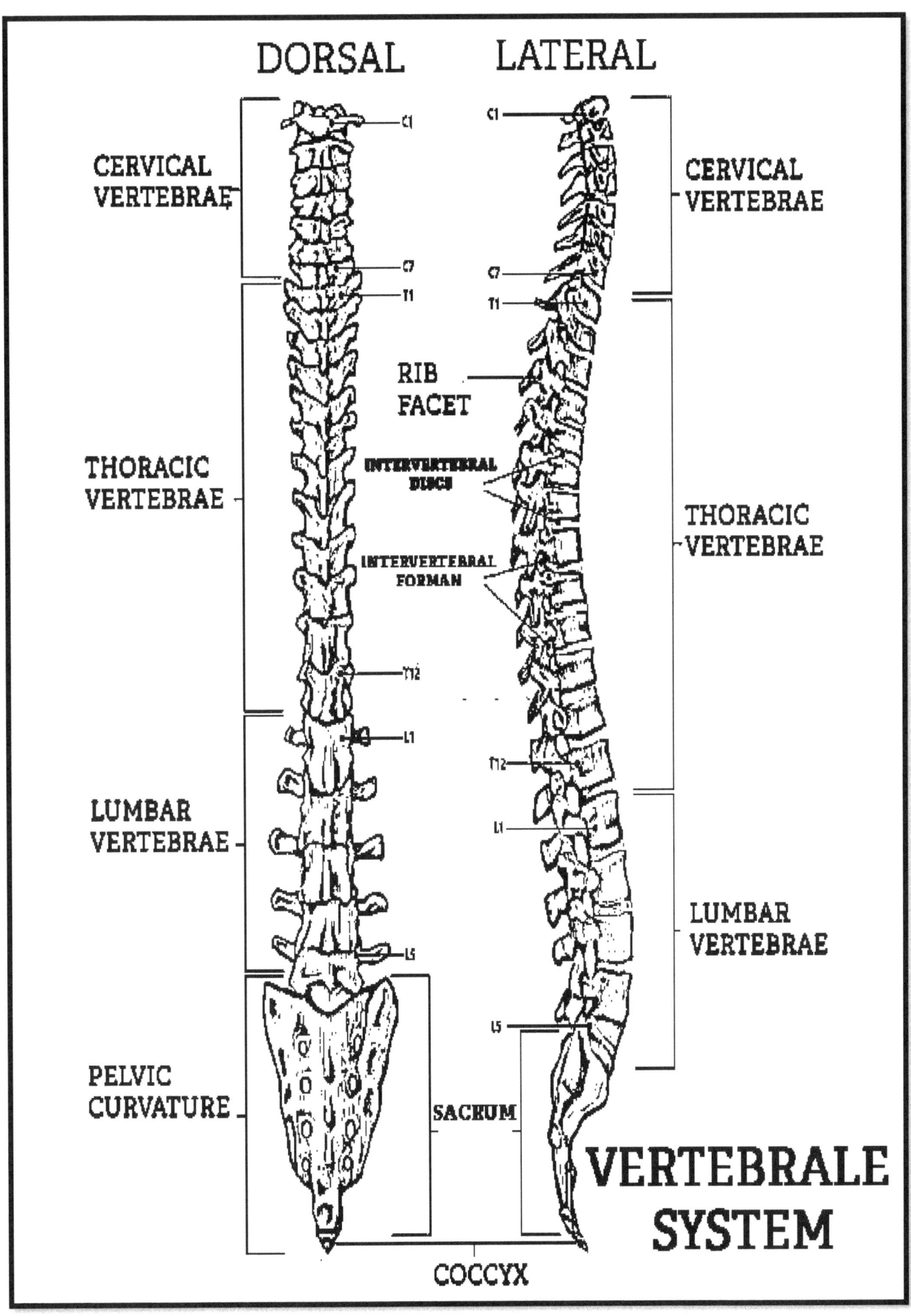

DORSAL   LATERAL

CERVICAL VERTEBRAE

CERVICAL VERTEBRAE

C1

C7

T1

RIB FACET

INTERVERTEBRAL DISCS

INTERVERTEBRAL FORMAN

THORACIC VERTEBRAE

THORACIC VERTEBRAE

T12

L1

LUMBAR VERTEBRAE

LUMBAR VERTEBRAE

T12

L1

L5

PELVIC CURVATURE

SACRUM

L5

COCCYX

VERTEBRALE SYSTEM

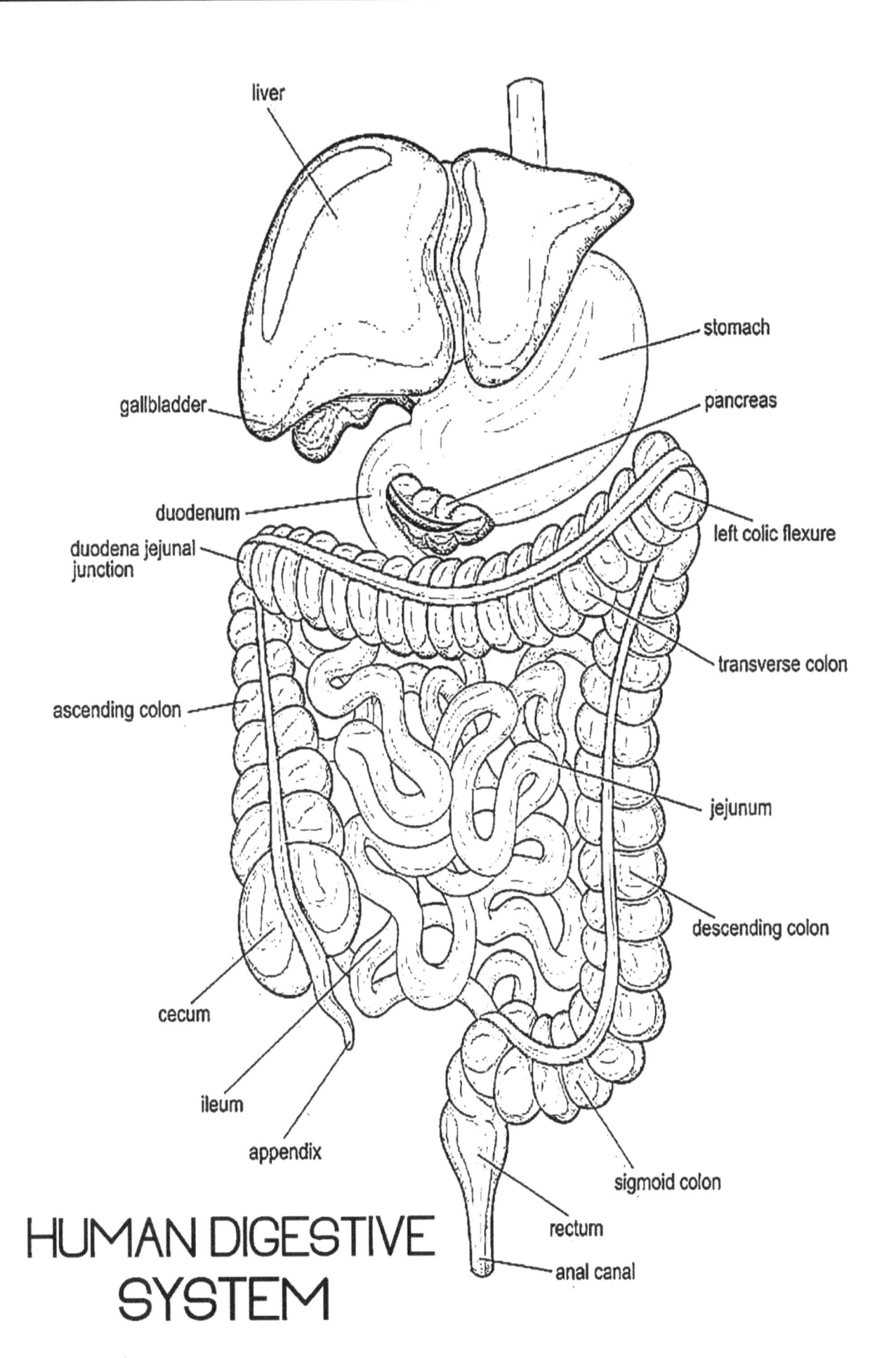

liver

stomach

gallbladder

pancreas

duodenum

left colic flexure

duodena jejunal junction

transverse colon

ascending colon

jejunum

descending colon

cecum

ileum

appendix

sigmoid colon

rectum

anal canal

HUMAN DIGESTIVE SYSTEM

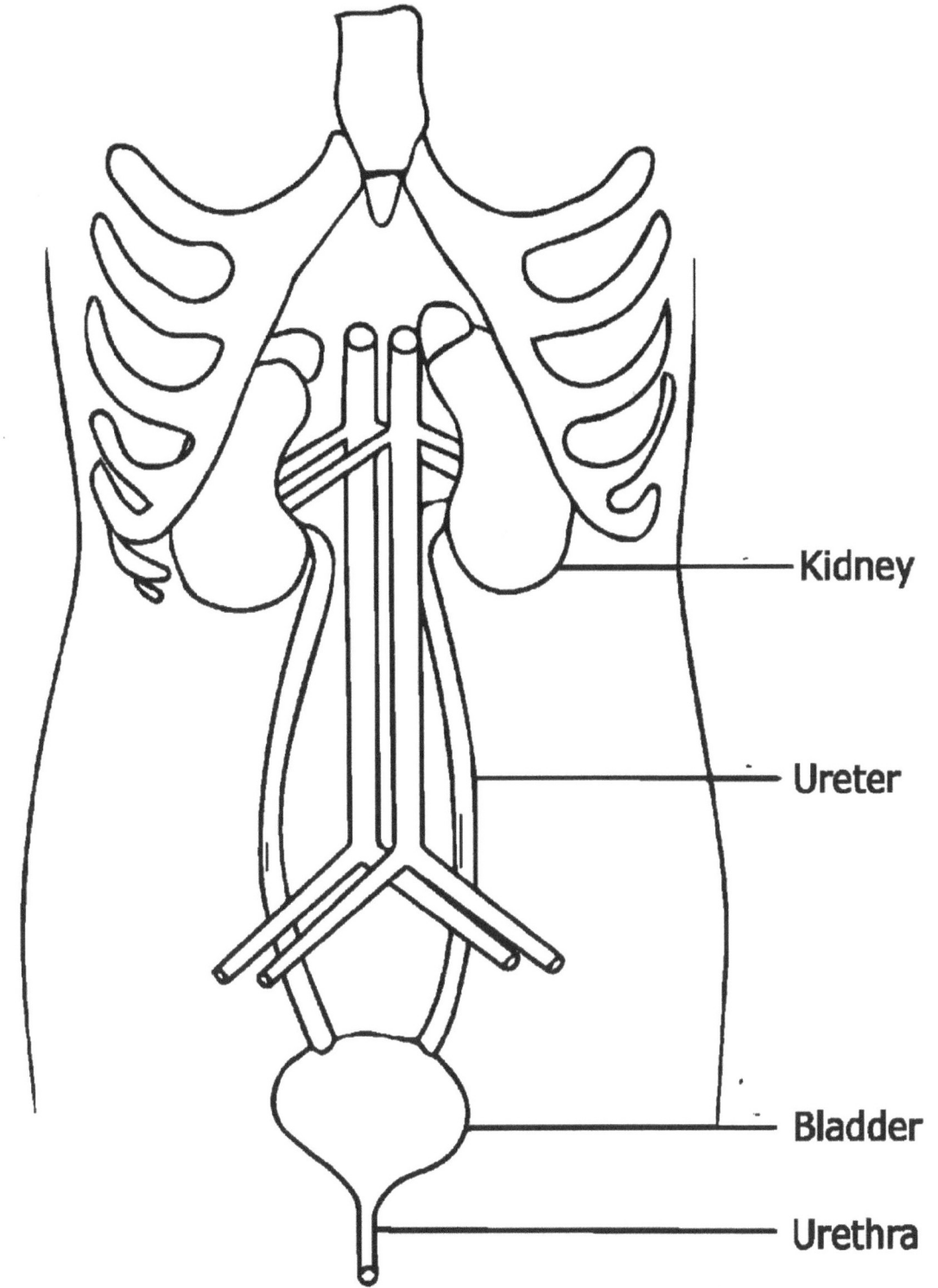

— Kidney

— Ureter

— Bladder

— Urethra

URINARY SYSTEM

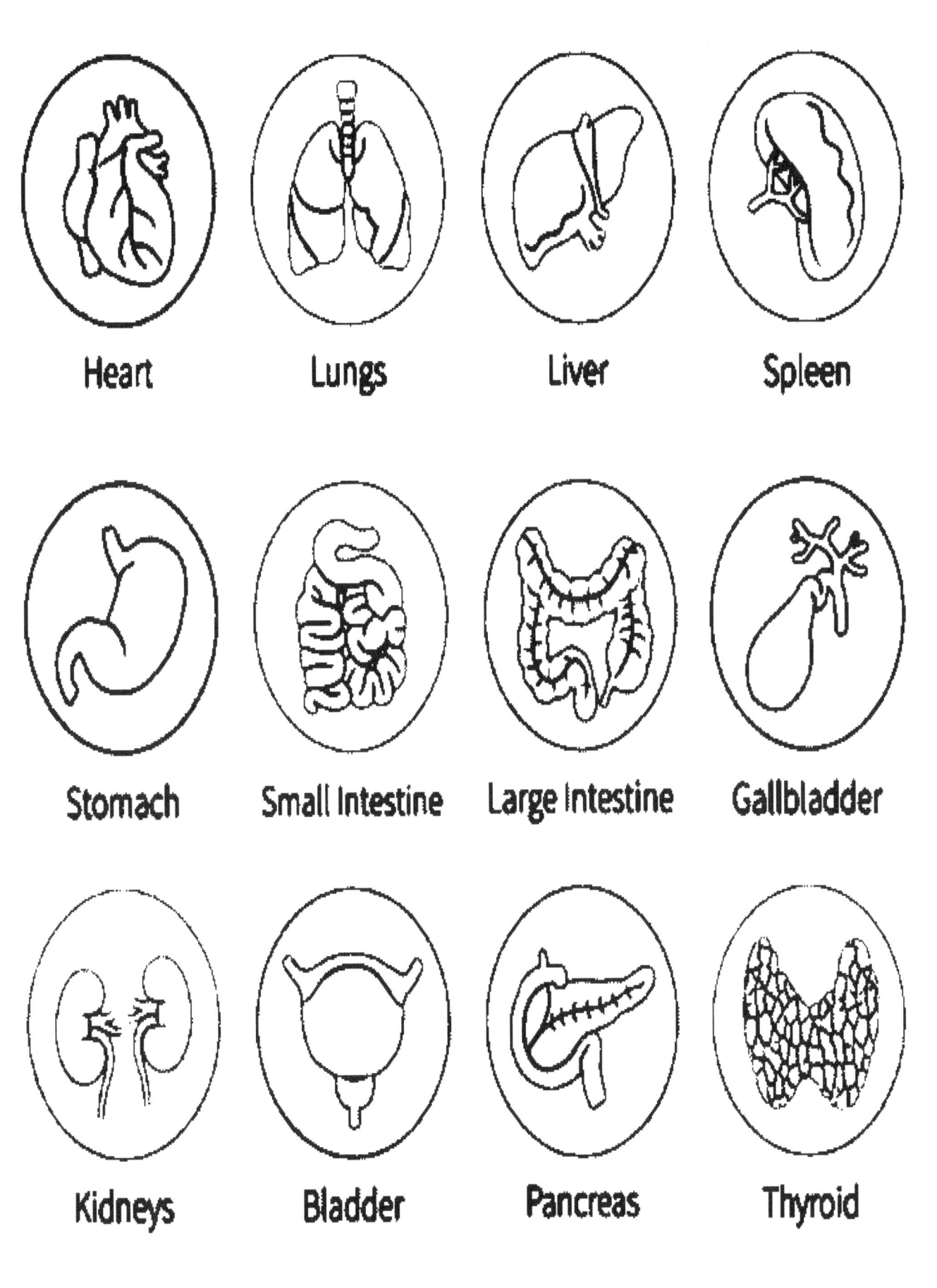

Heart   Lungs   Liver   Spleen

Stomach   Small Intestine   Large Intestine   Gallbladder

Kidneys   Bladder   Pancreas   Thyroid

COLOR EACH ORGAN

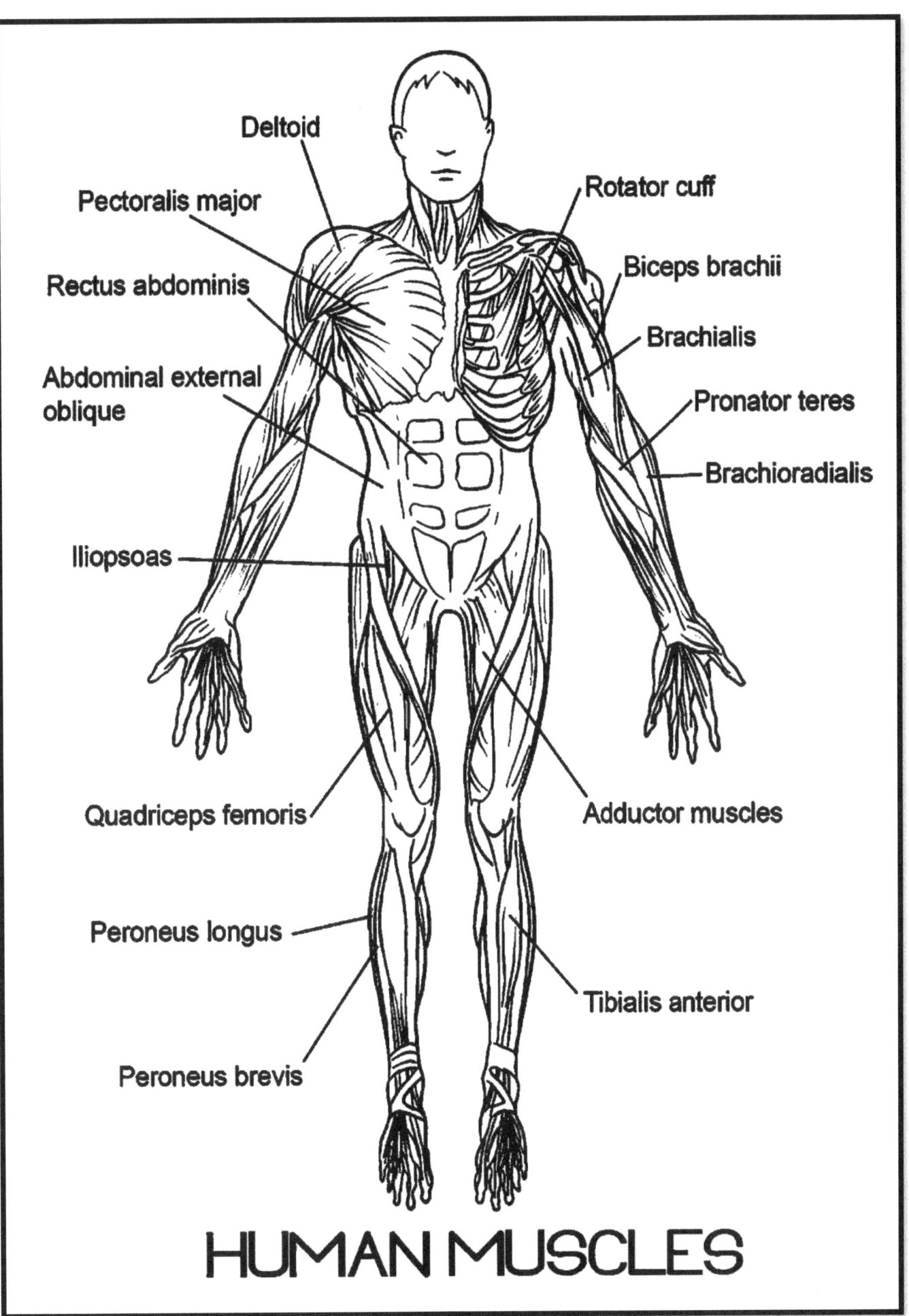

Deltoid

Pectoralis major

Rectus abdominis

Abdominal external oblique

Iliopsoas

Quadriceps femoris

Peroneus longus

Peroneus brevis

Rotator cuff

Biceps brachii

Brachialis

Pronator teres

Brachioradialis

Adductor muscles

Tibialis anterior

HUMAN MUSCLES

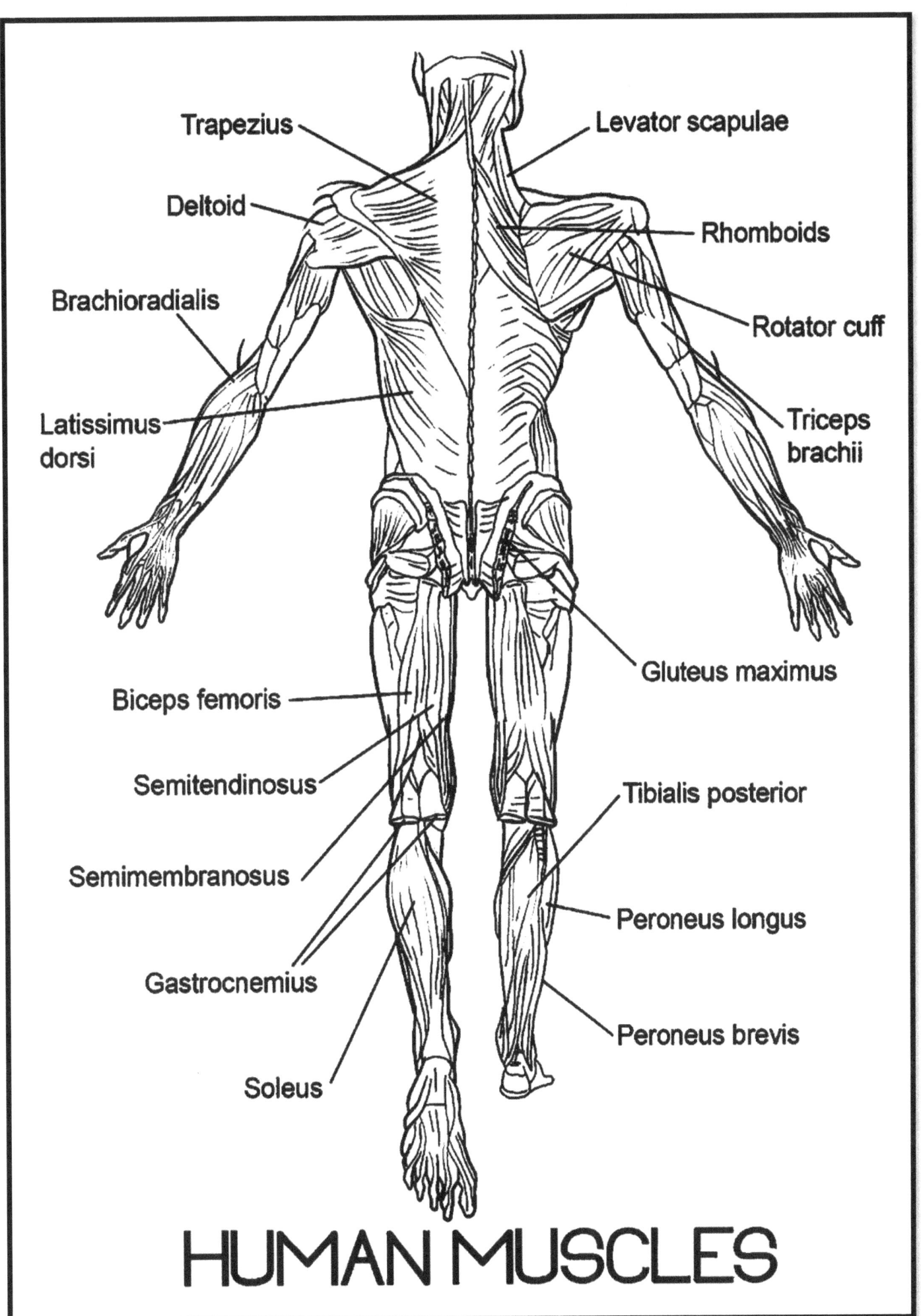

Trapezius

Levator scapulae

Deltoid

Rhomboids

Brachioradialis

Rotator cuff

Latissimus dorsi

Triceps brachii

Gluteus maximus

Biceps femoris

Semitendinosus

Tibialis posterior

Semimembranosus

Peroneus longus

Gastrocnemius

Peroneus brevis

Soleus

HUMAN MUSCLES

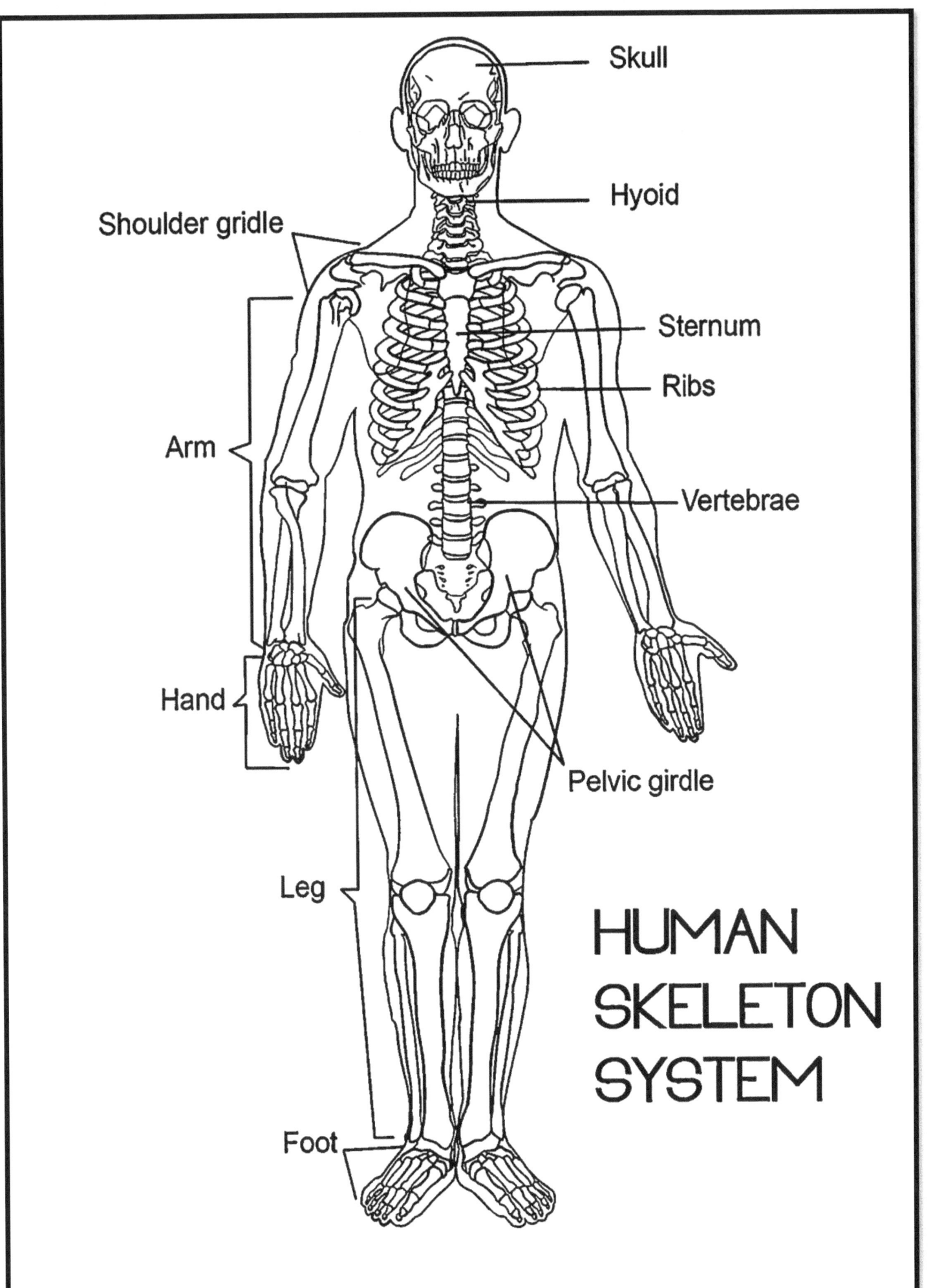

Skull

Hyoid

Shoulder gridle

Sternum

Ribs

Arm

Vertebrae

Hand

Pelvic girdle

Leg

HUMAN
SKELETON
SYSTEM

Foot

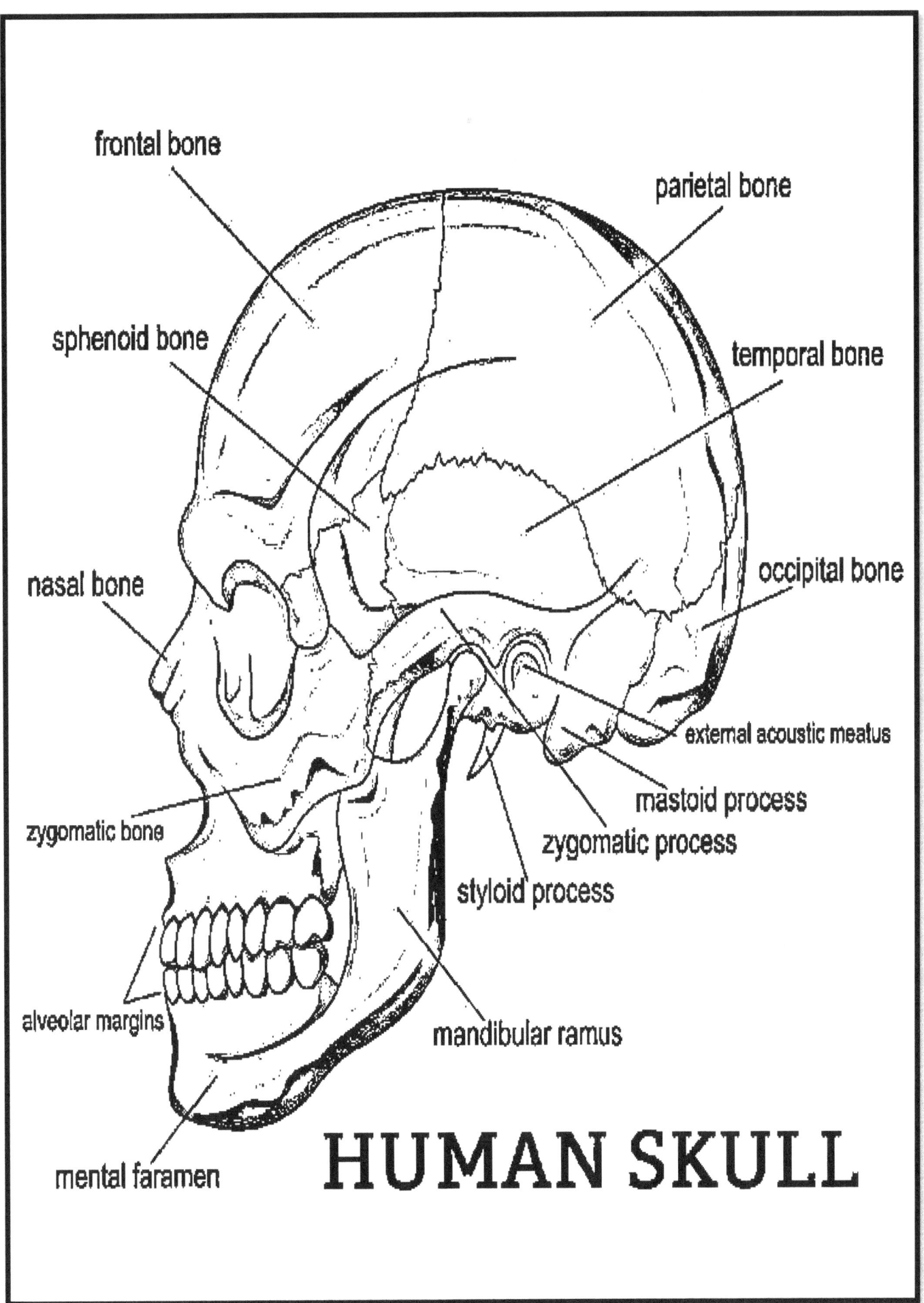

frontal bone

parietal bone

sphenoid bone

temporal bone

nasal bone

occipital bone

external acoustic meatus

mastoid process

zygomatic bone

zygomatic process

styloid process

alveolar margins

mandibular ramus

mental faramen

HUMAN SKULL

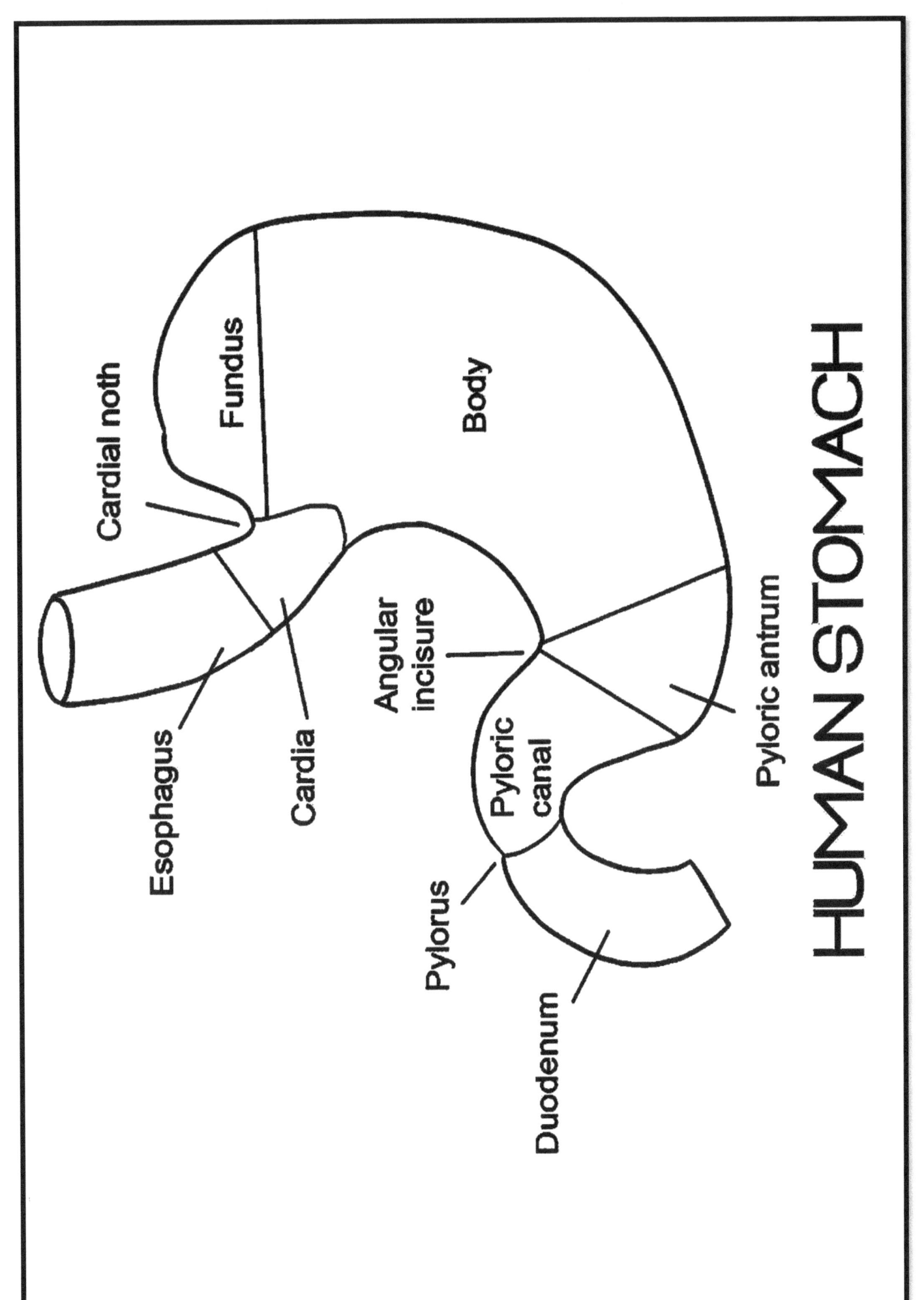

HUMAN STOMACH

Cardial noth

Fundus

Body

Esophagus

Cardia

Angular incisure

Pyloric canal

Pylorus

Duodenum

Pyloric antrum

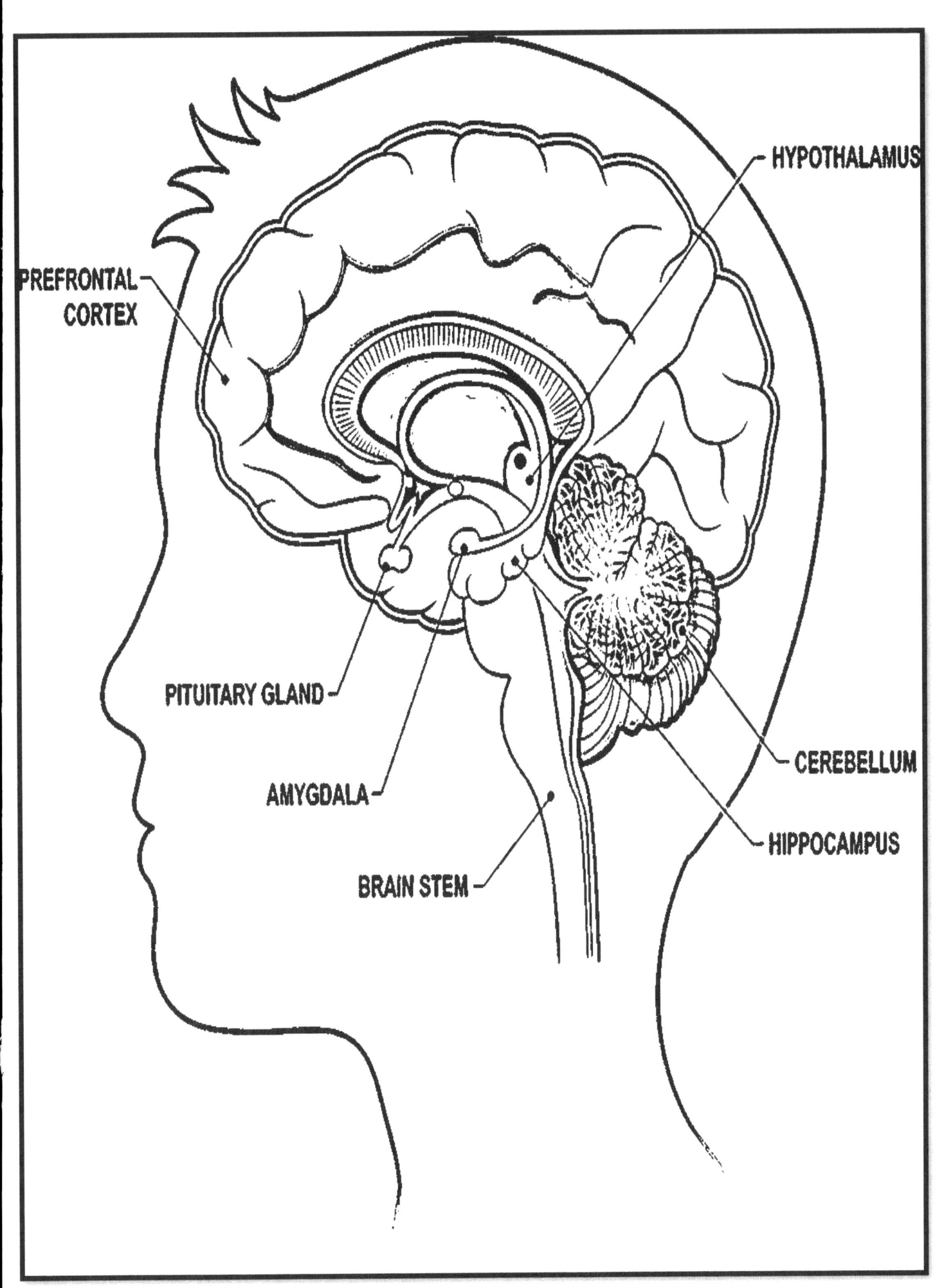

HYPOTHALAMUS

PREFRONTAL
CORTEX

PITUITARY GLAND

AMYGDALA

BRAIN STEM

CEREBELLUM

HIPPOCAMPUS

BRAIN ANATOMY

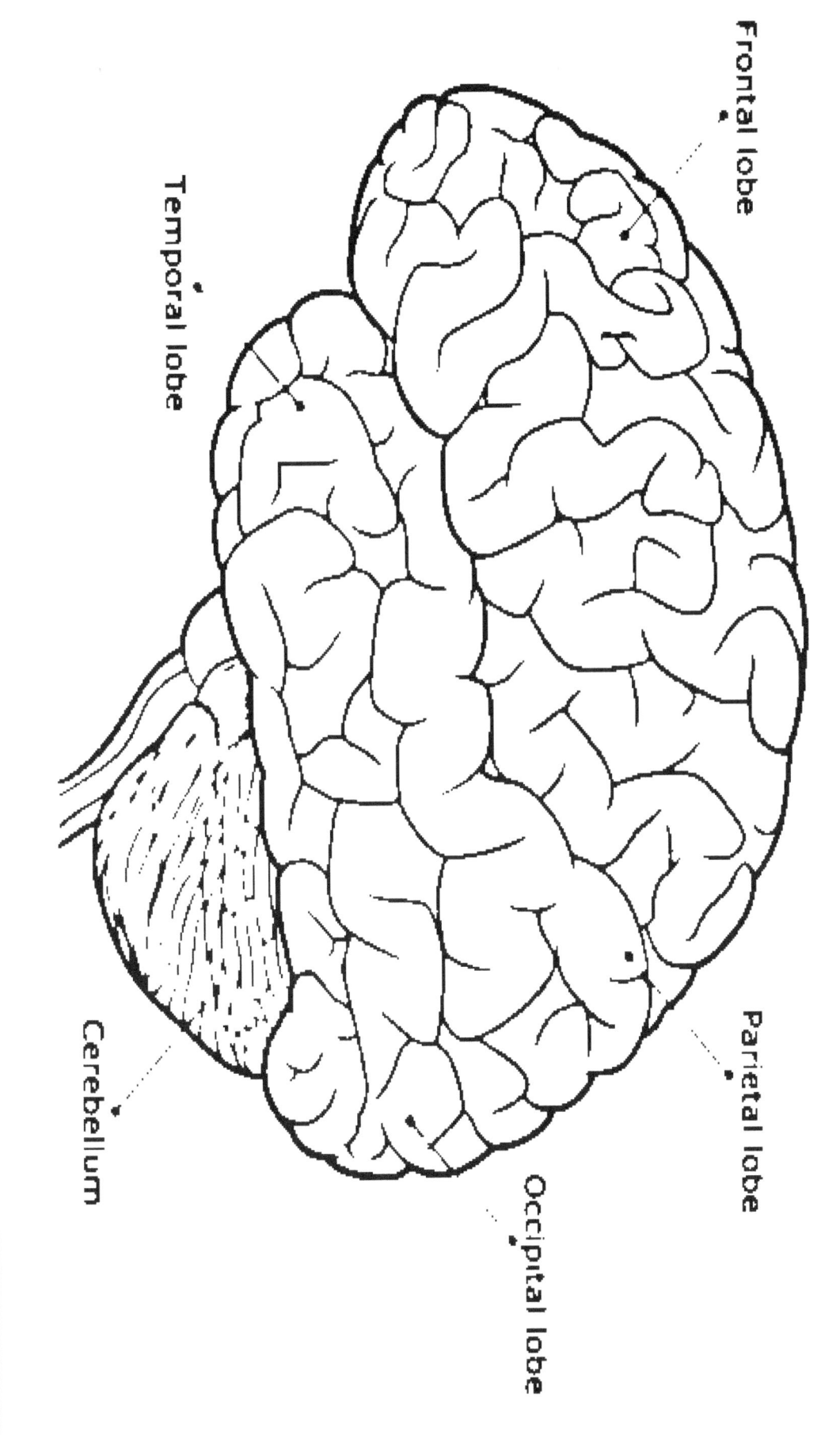

Frontal lobe

Temporal lobe

Cerebellum

Parietal lobe

Occipital lobe

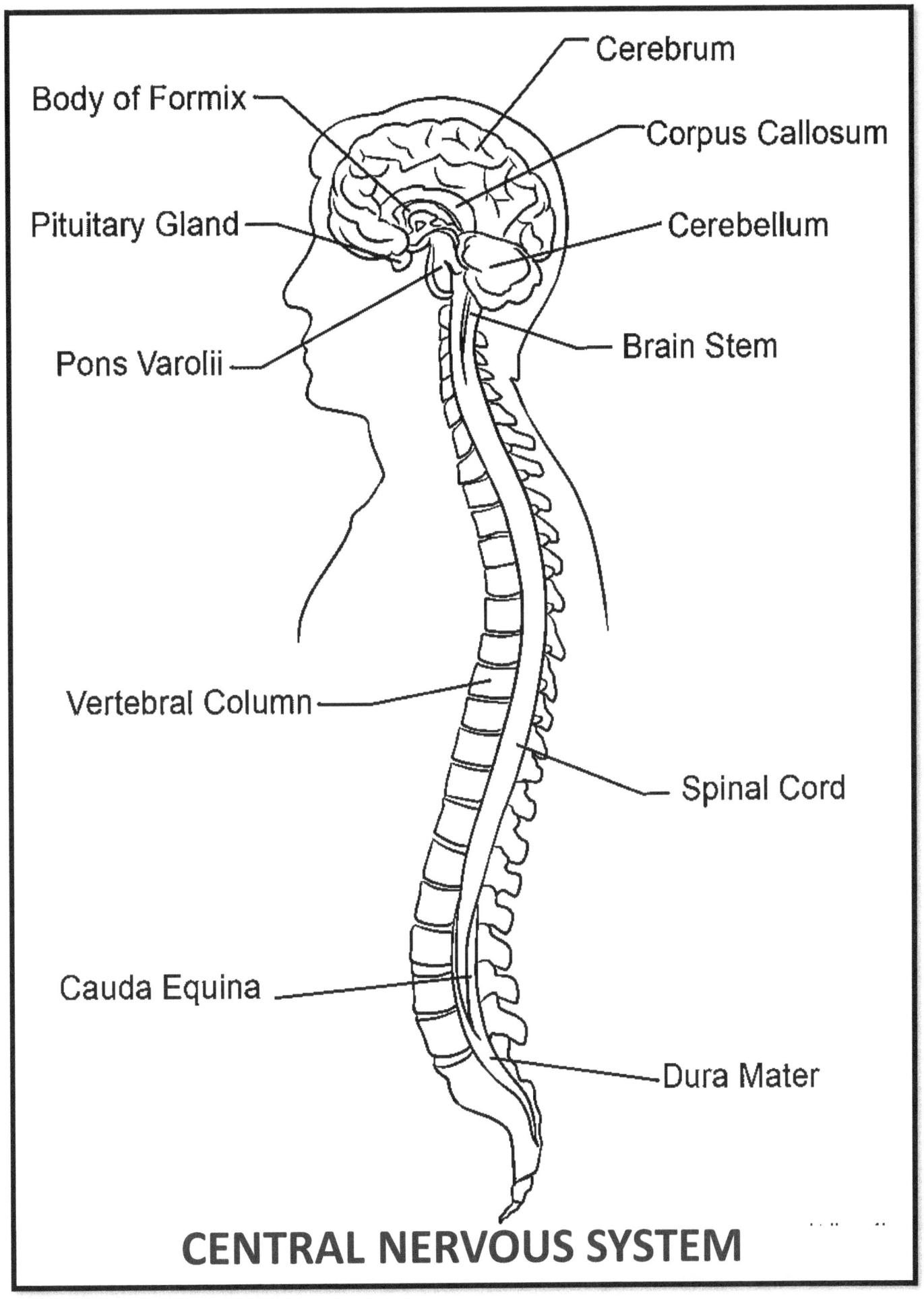

Cerebrum

Body of Formix

Corpus Callosum

Pituitary Gland

Cerebellum

Pons Varolii

Brain Stem

Vertebral Column

Spinal Cord

Cauda Equina

Dura Mater

CENTRAL NERVOUS SYSTEM

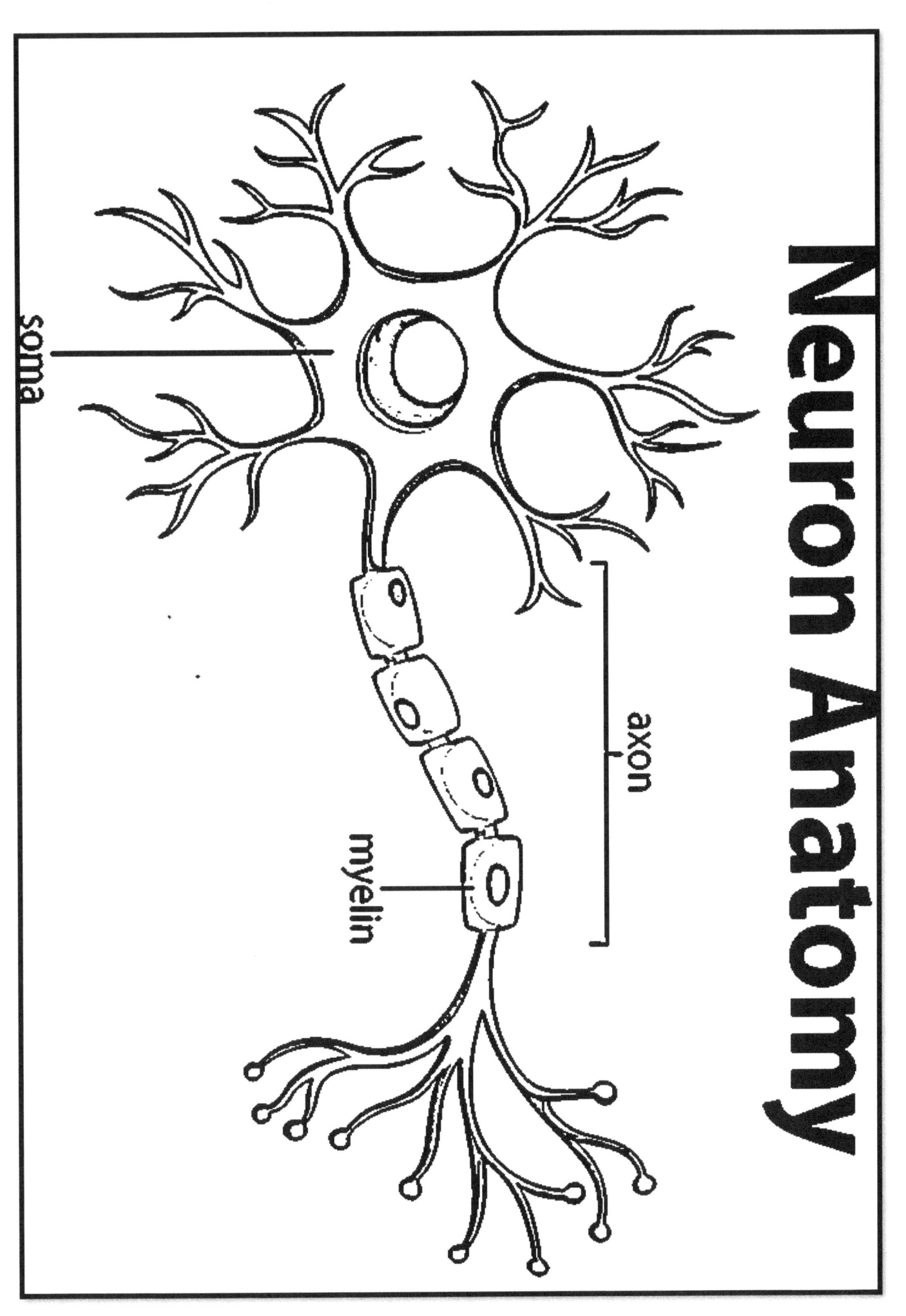

Neuron Anatomy

soma

axon

myelin

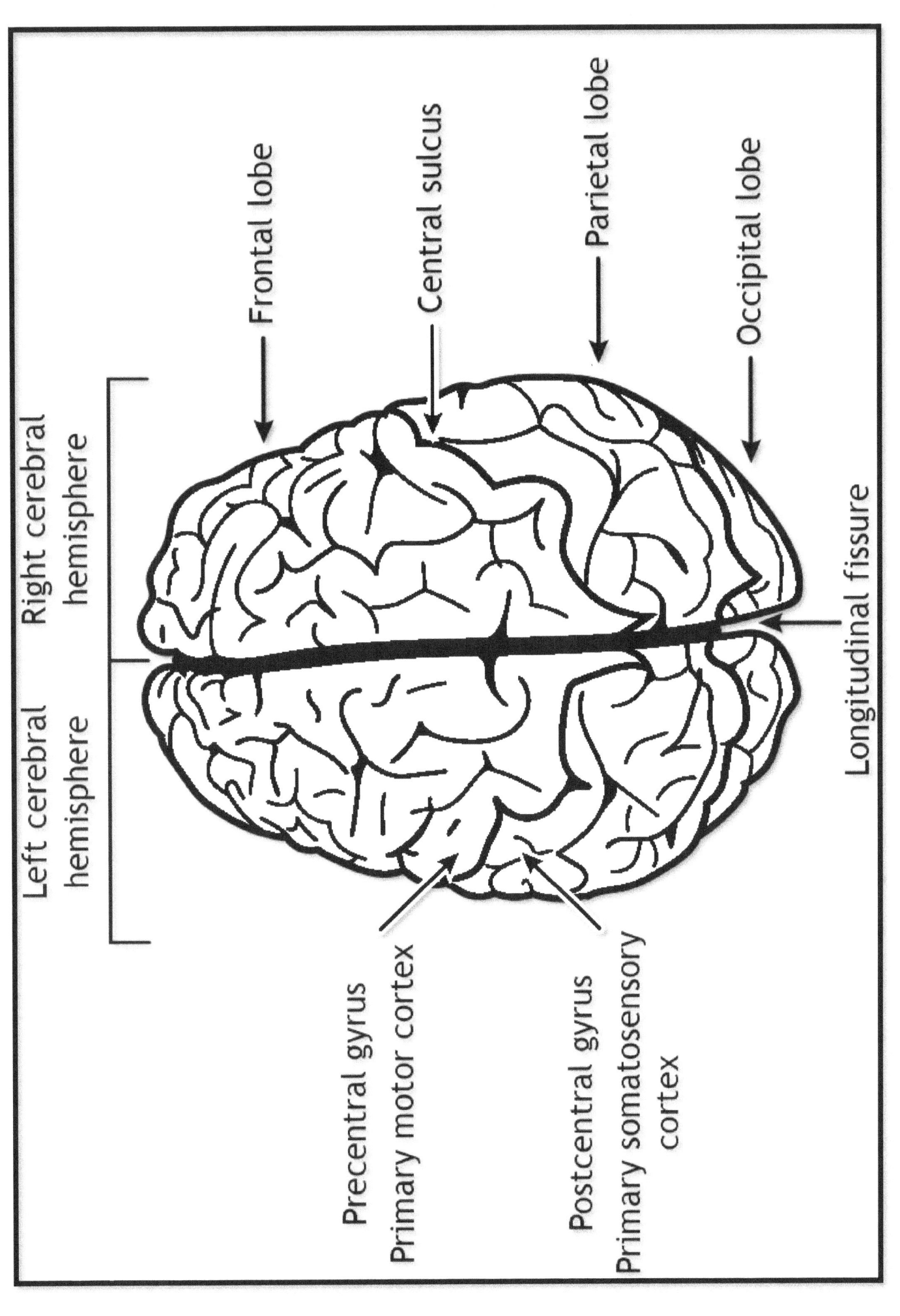

LIMBIC SYSTEM

Corpus callosum

Interthalamic adhesion

Fornix

Thalamus

Occipital lobe

Cingulate gyrus

Cerebellum

Choroid plexus

Anterior group of thalamic nuclei

Frontal lobe

Cingulate gyrus

Hypothalamus

Amygdala

Mamillary body

Hippocampus

Brain stem

BRAIN STEM

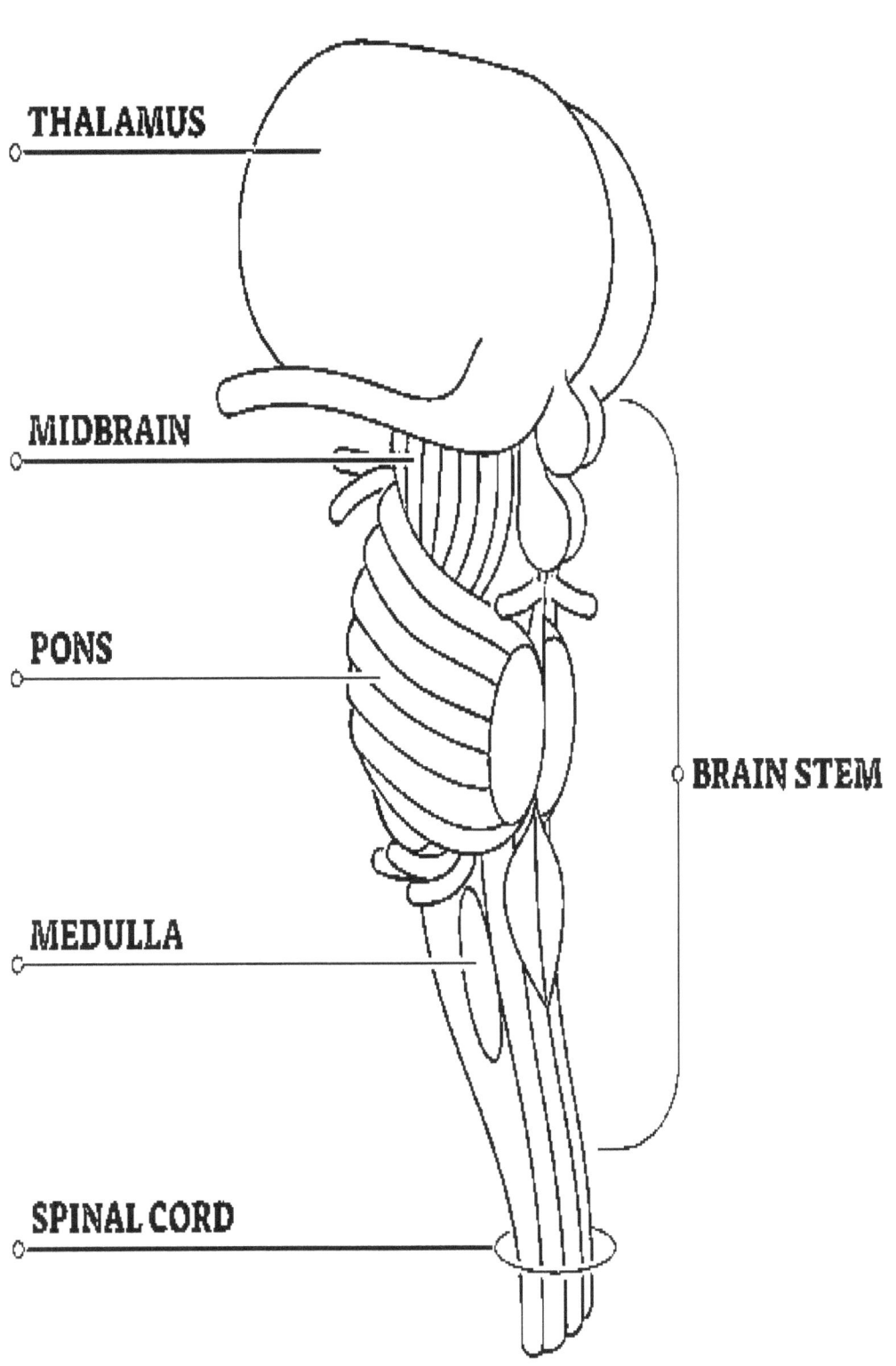

THALAMUS

MIDBRAIN

PONS

MEDULLA

SPINAL CORD

BRAIN STEM

STROKE

BRAIN

Blood Clot

Affected Area

Blood Flow

Artery

BRAIN STIMULATION

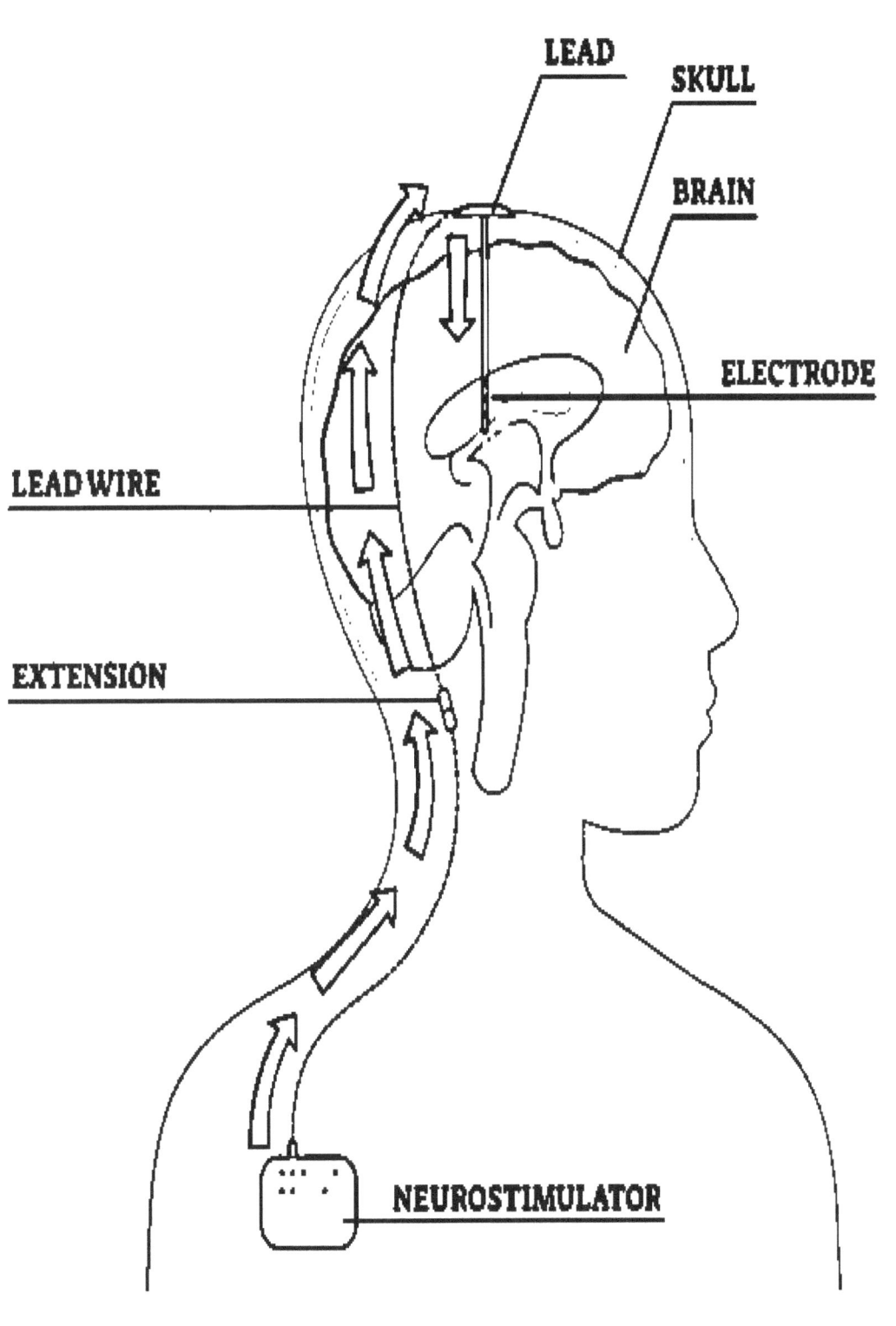

LEAD

SKULL

BRAIN

ELECTRODE

LEAD WIRE

EXTENSION

NEUROSTIMULATOR

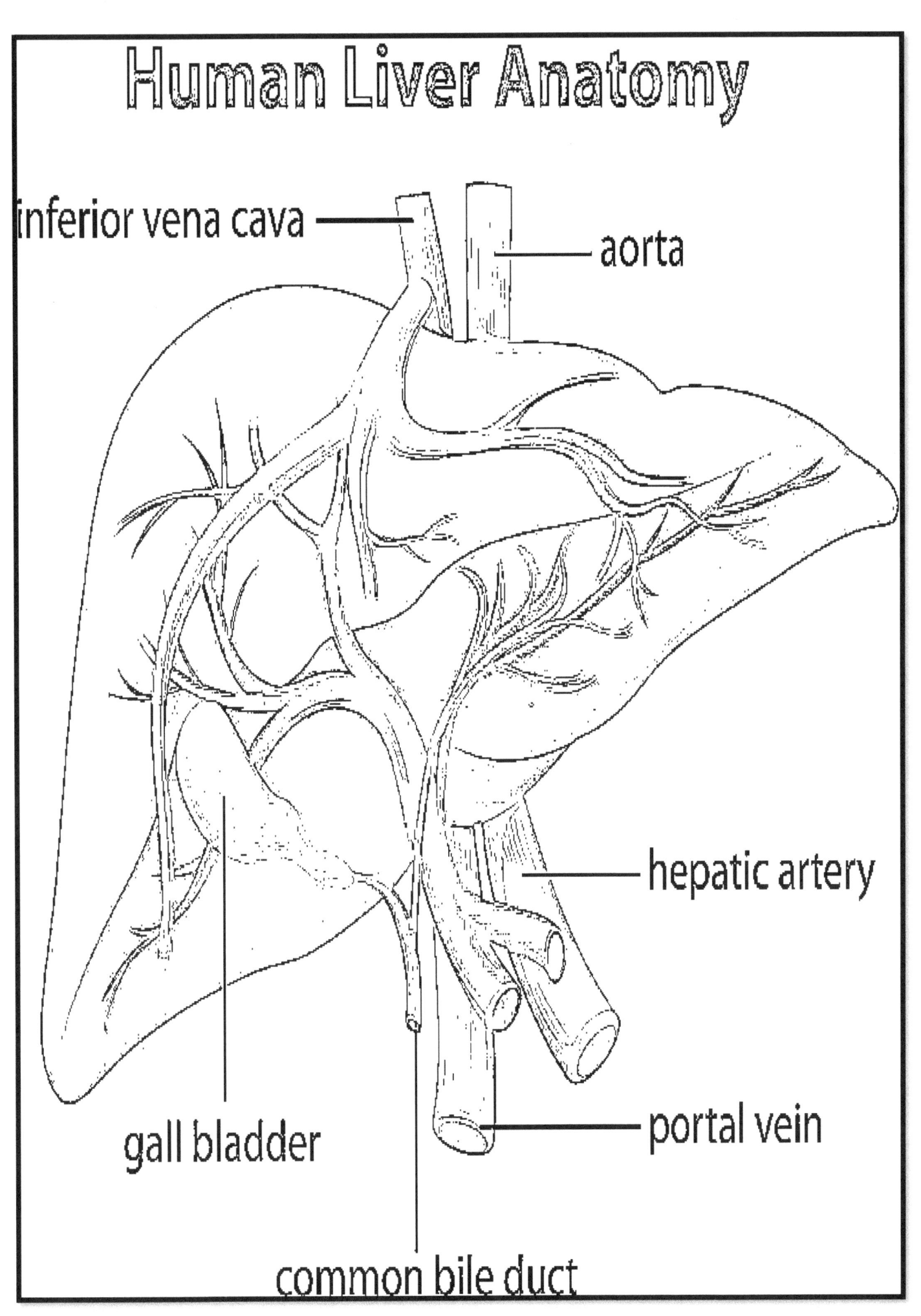

Human Liver Anatomy

inferior vena cava

aorta

hepatic artery

gall bladder

portal vein

common bile duct

THE HUMAN KNEE

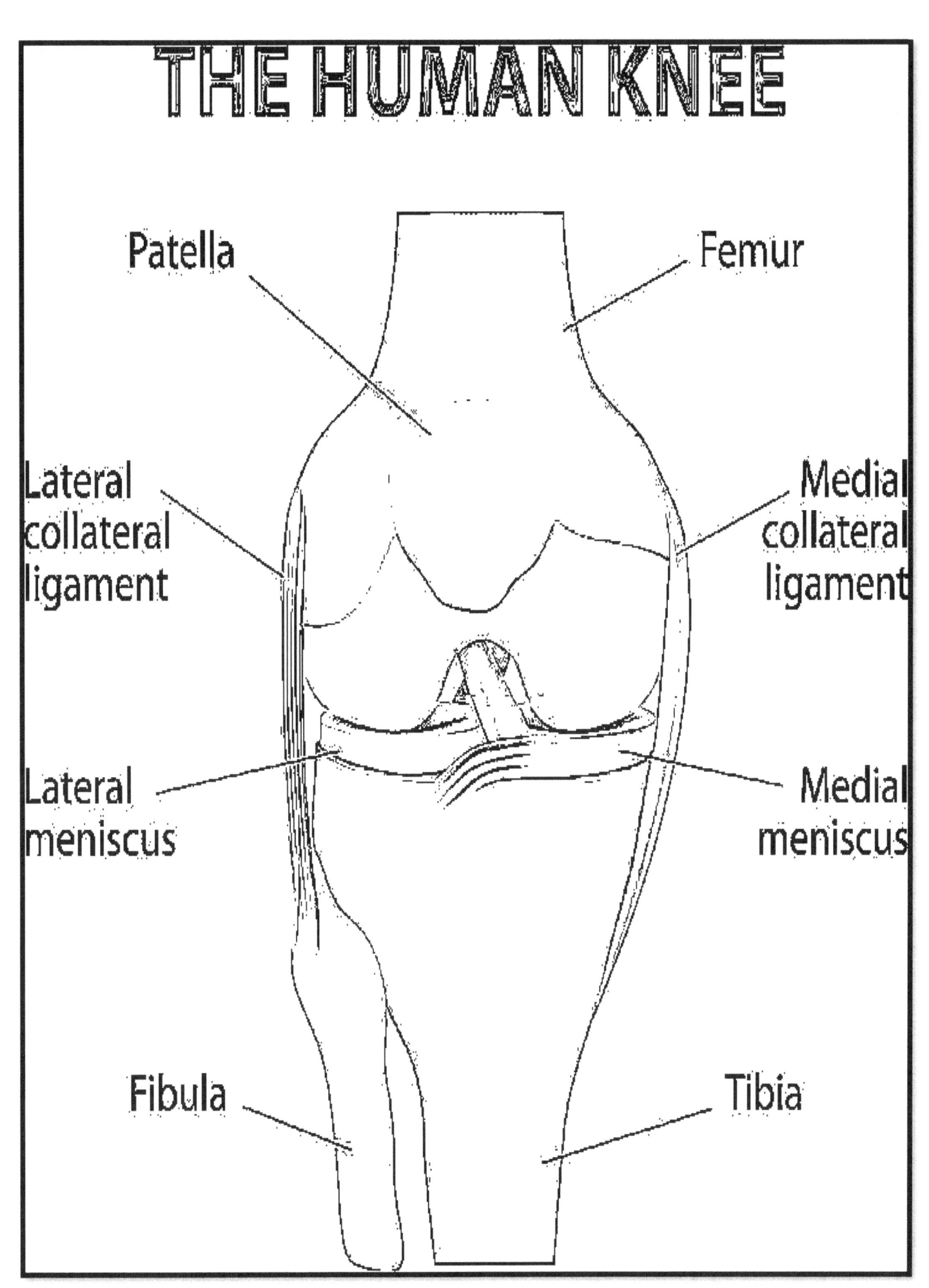

Patella

Femur

Lateral collateral ligament

Medial collateral ligament

Lateral meniscus

Medial meniscus

Fibula

Tibia

HUMAN TONGUE
the organg of taste

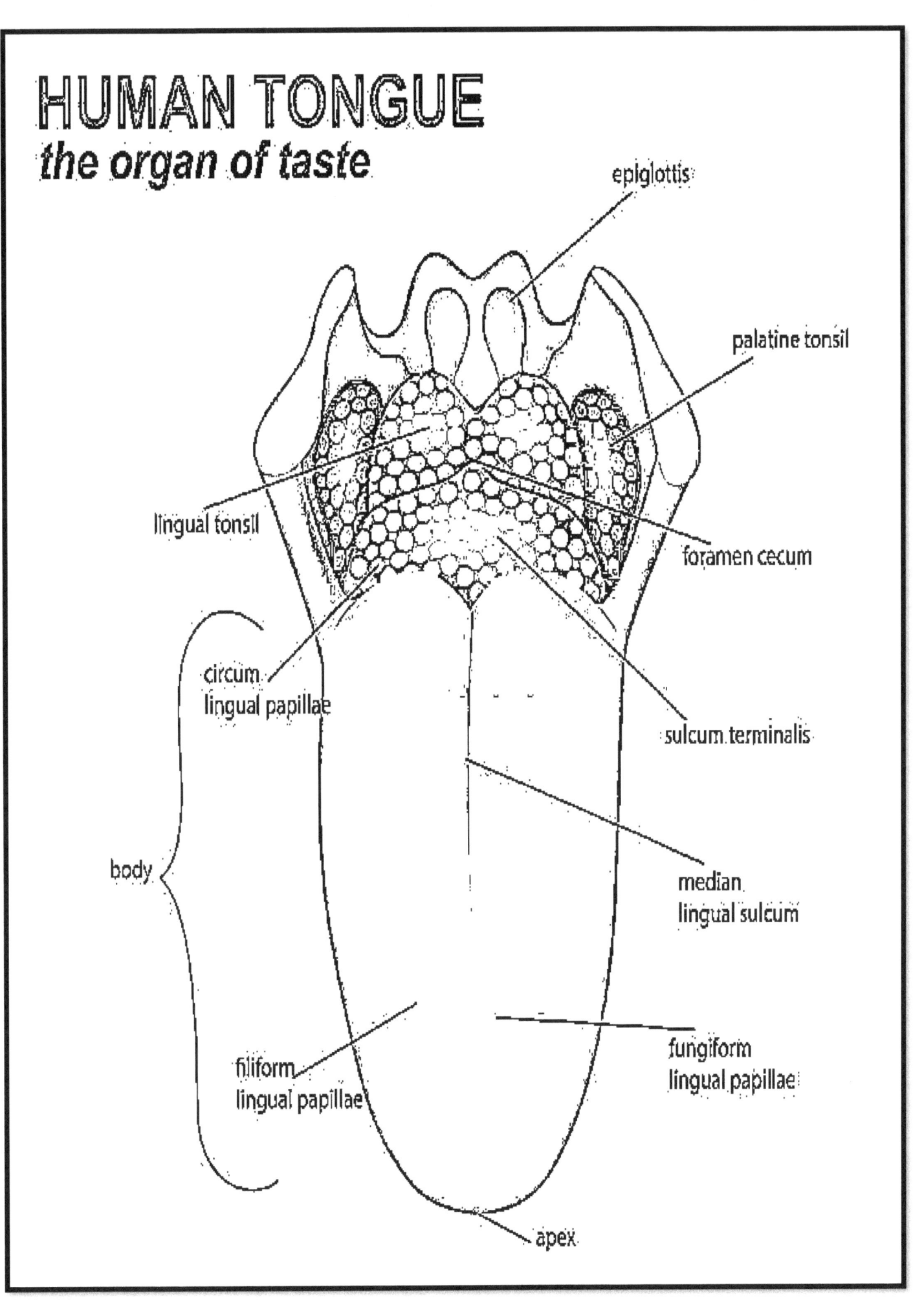

epiglottis

palatine tonsil

lingual tonsil

foramen cecum

circum lingual papillae

sulcum terminalis

body

median lingual sulcum

filiform lingual papillae

fungiform lingual papillae

apex

ANATOMY OF ANAL CANAL

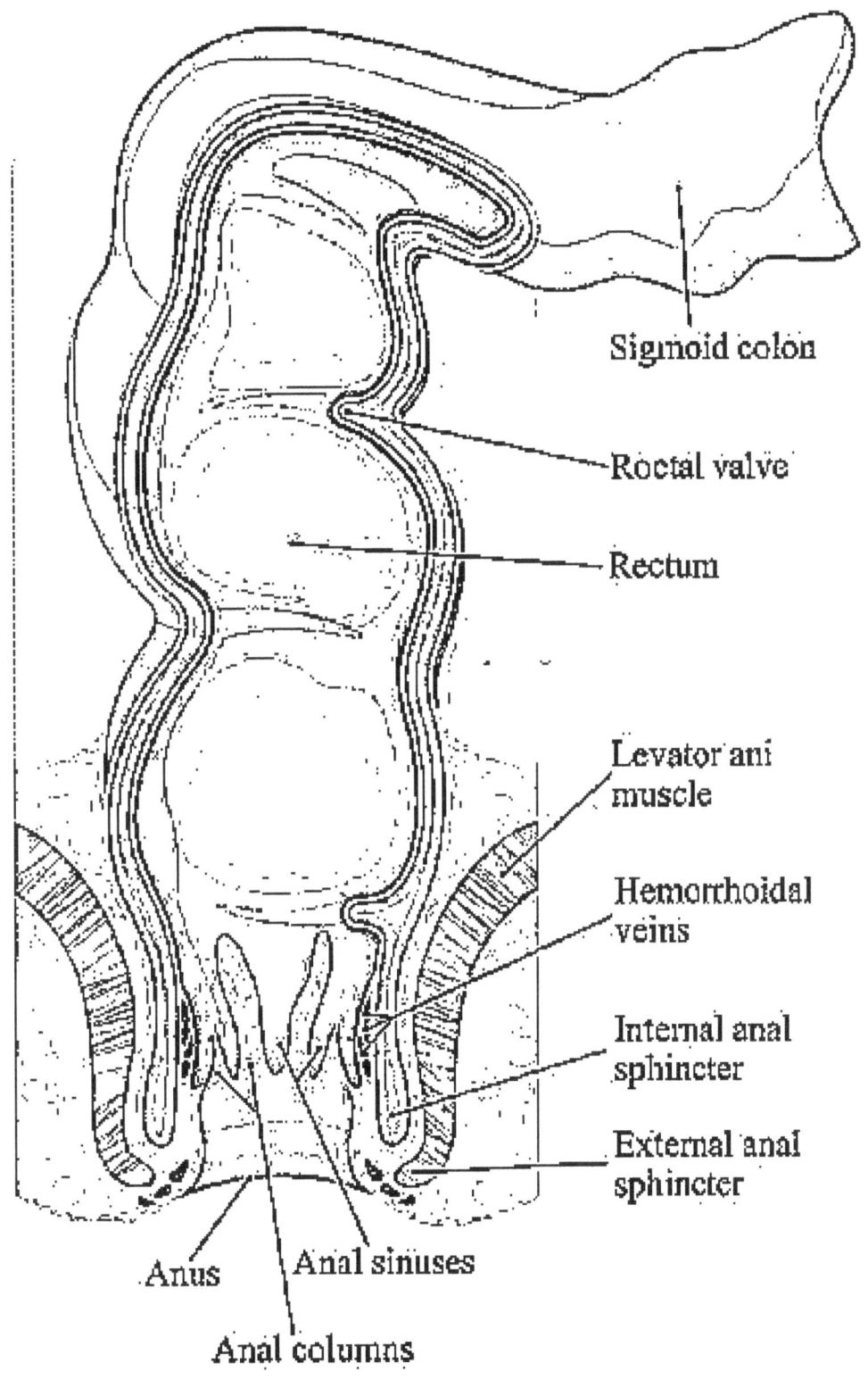

Sigmoid colon

Rectal valve

Rectum

Levator ani muscle

Hemorrhoidal veins

Internal anal sphincter

External anal sphincter

Anus

Anal sinuses

Anal columns

Bones of the Hand

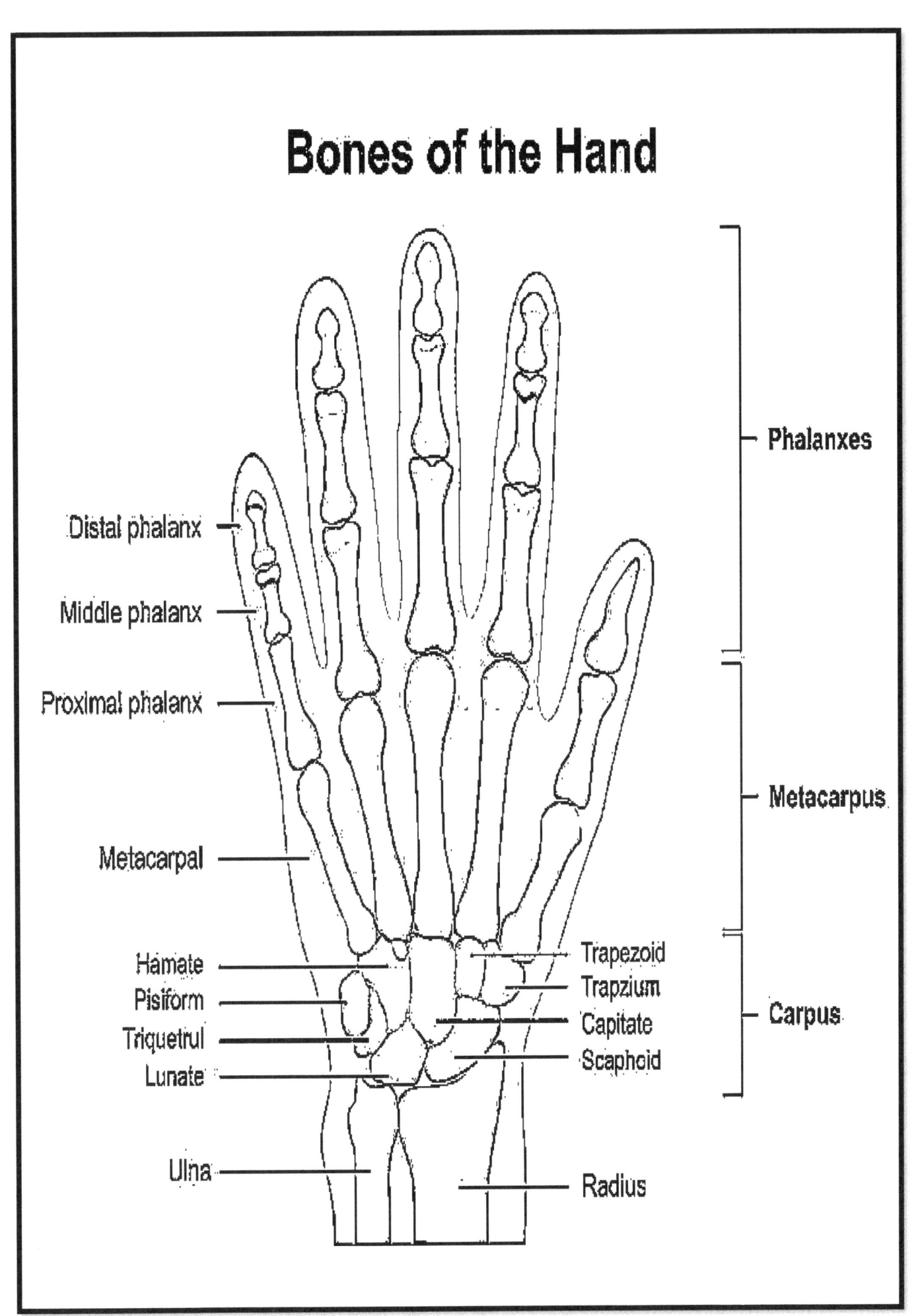

Phalanxes

Distal phalanx

Middle phalanx

Proximal phalanx

Metacarpus

Metacarpal

Hamate — Trapezoid
Pisiform — Trapzium
Triquetrul — Capitate
Lunate — Scaphoid

Carpus

Ulna — Radius

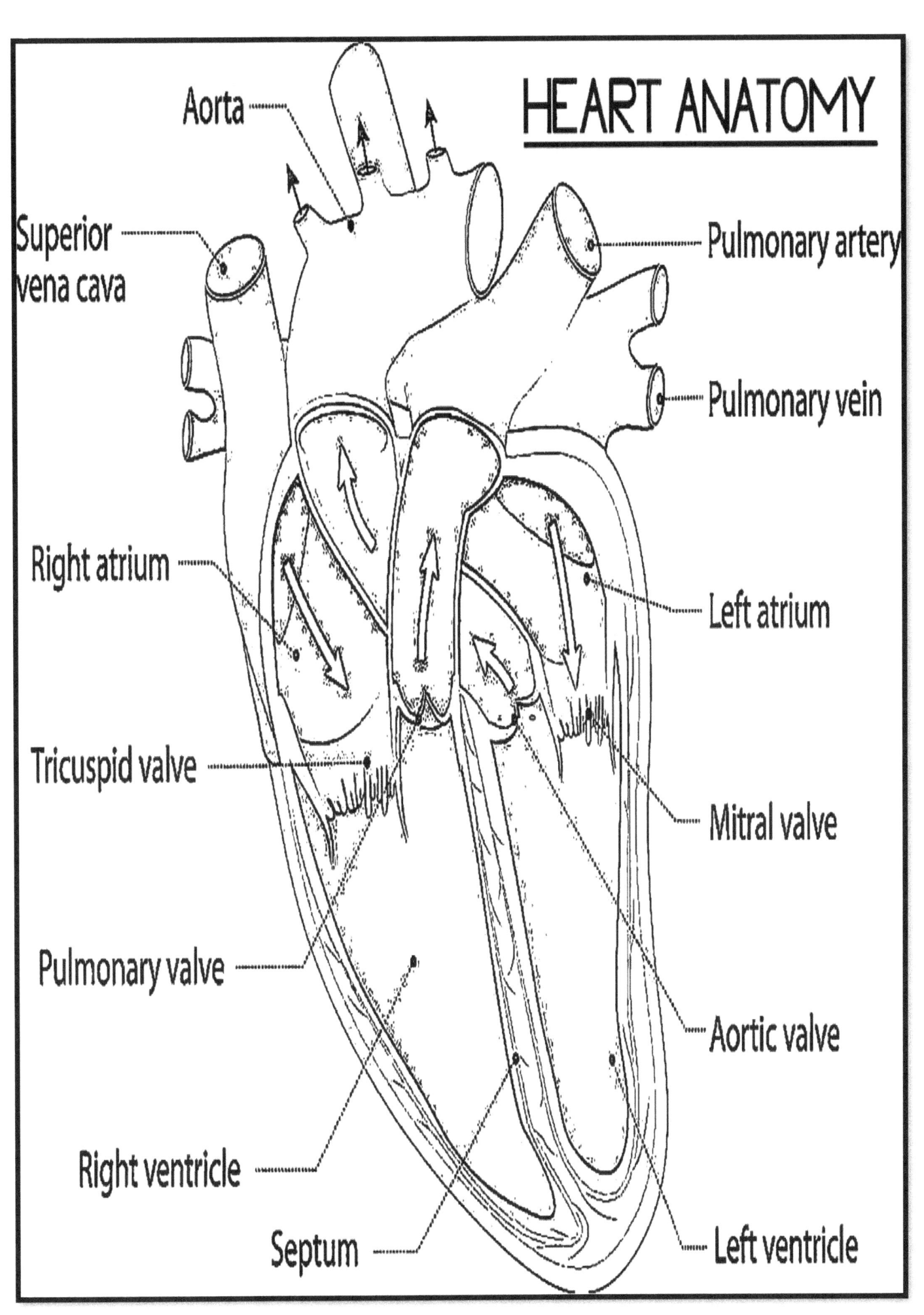

HEART ANATOMY

Aorta

Superior vena cava

Pulmonary artery

Pulmonary vein

Right atrium

Left atrium

Tricuspid valve

Mitral valve

Pulmonary valve

Aortic valve

Right ventricle

Septum

Left ventricle

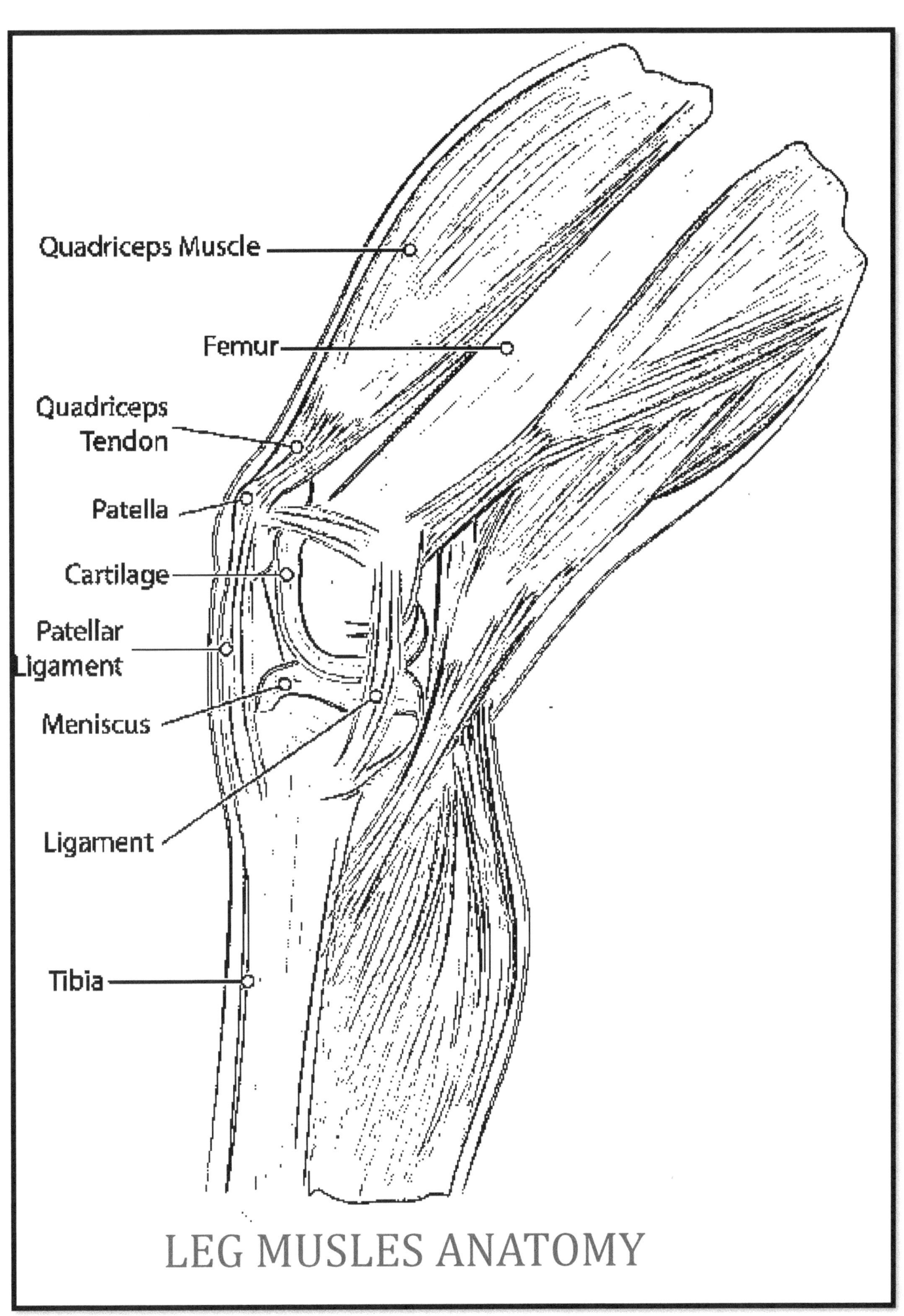

Quadriceps Muscle

Femur

Quadriceps
Tendon

Patella

Cartilage

Patellar
Ligament

Meniscus

Ligament

Tibia

LEG MUSLES ANATOMY

TOOTH ANATOMY

Enamal

Dentin

Pulp

Gum

Root canal

Root-end opening

Crown

Root

Bone

Blood Vessels

HAIR ANATOMY

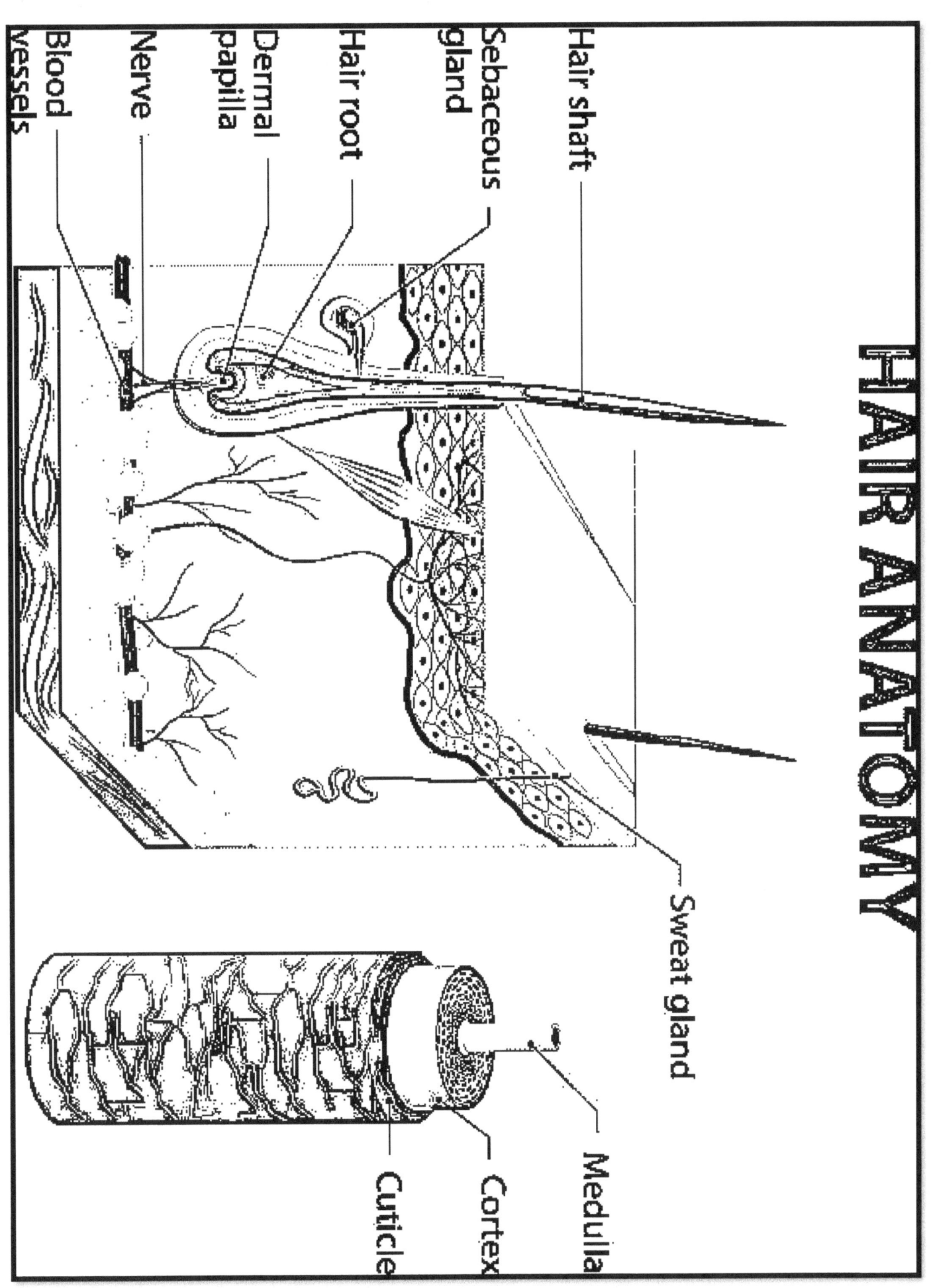

Blood
vessels

Nerve

Dermal
papilla

Hair root

Sebaceous
gland

Hair shaft

Sweat gland

Cuticle

Cortex

Medulla

STRUCTURE OF THE SKIN

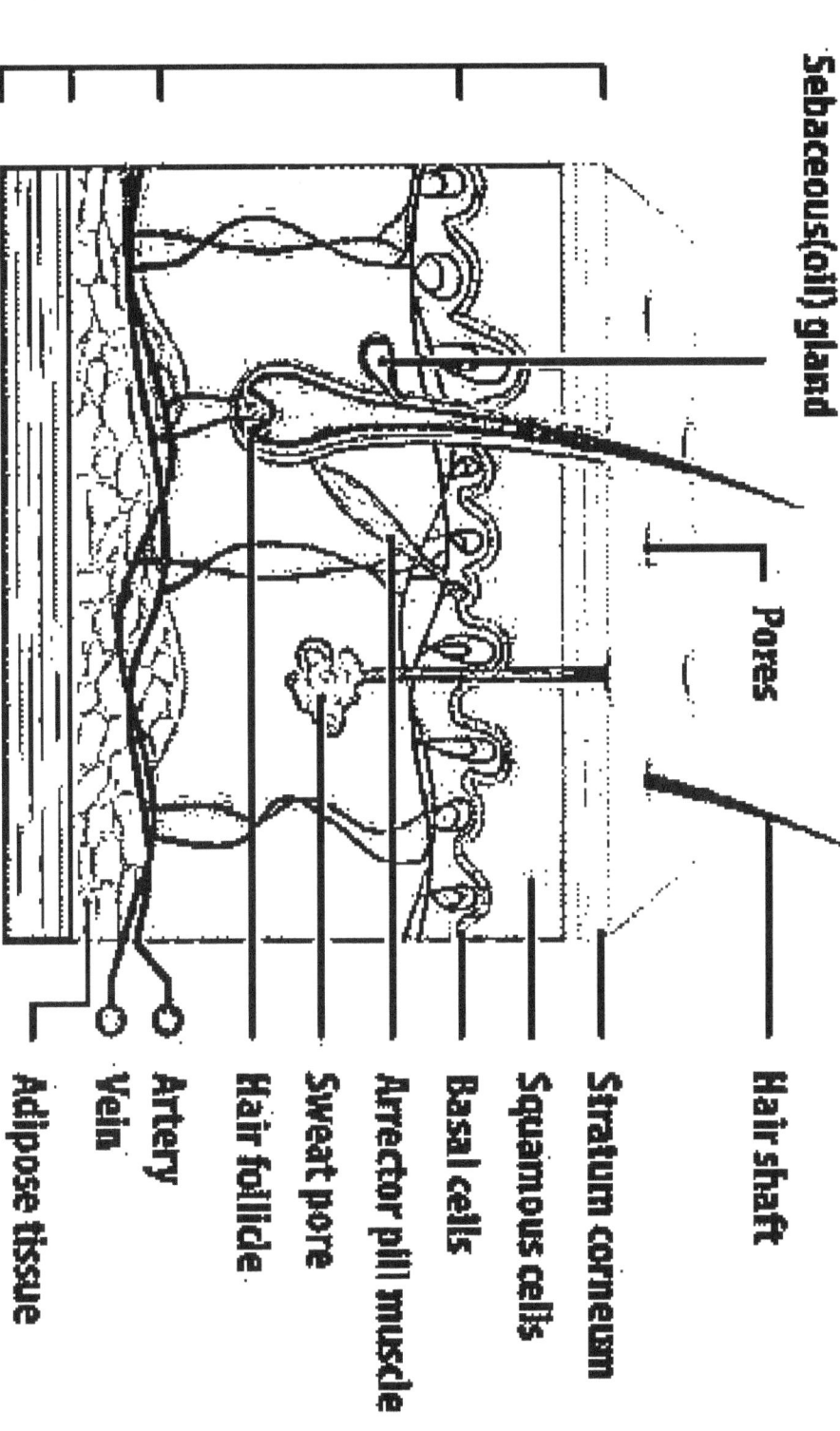

Epidermis

Dermis

Hypodermis
(Subcutaneous tissue)

Muscle

Sebaceous(oil) gland

Pores

Hair shaft

Stratum corneum

Squamous cells

Basal cells

Arrector pili muscle

Sweat pore

Hair follicle

Artery

Vein

Adipose tissue

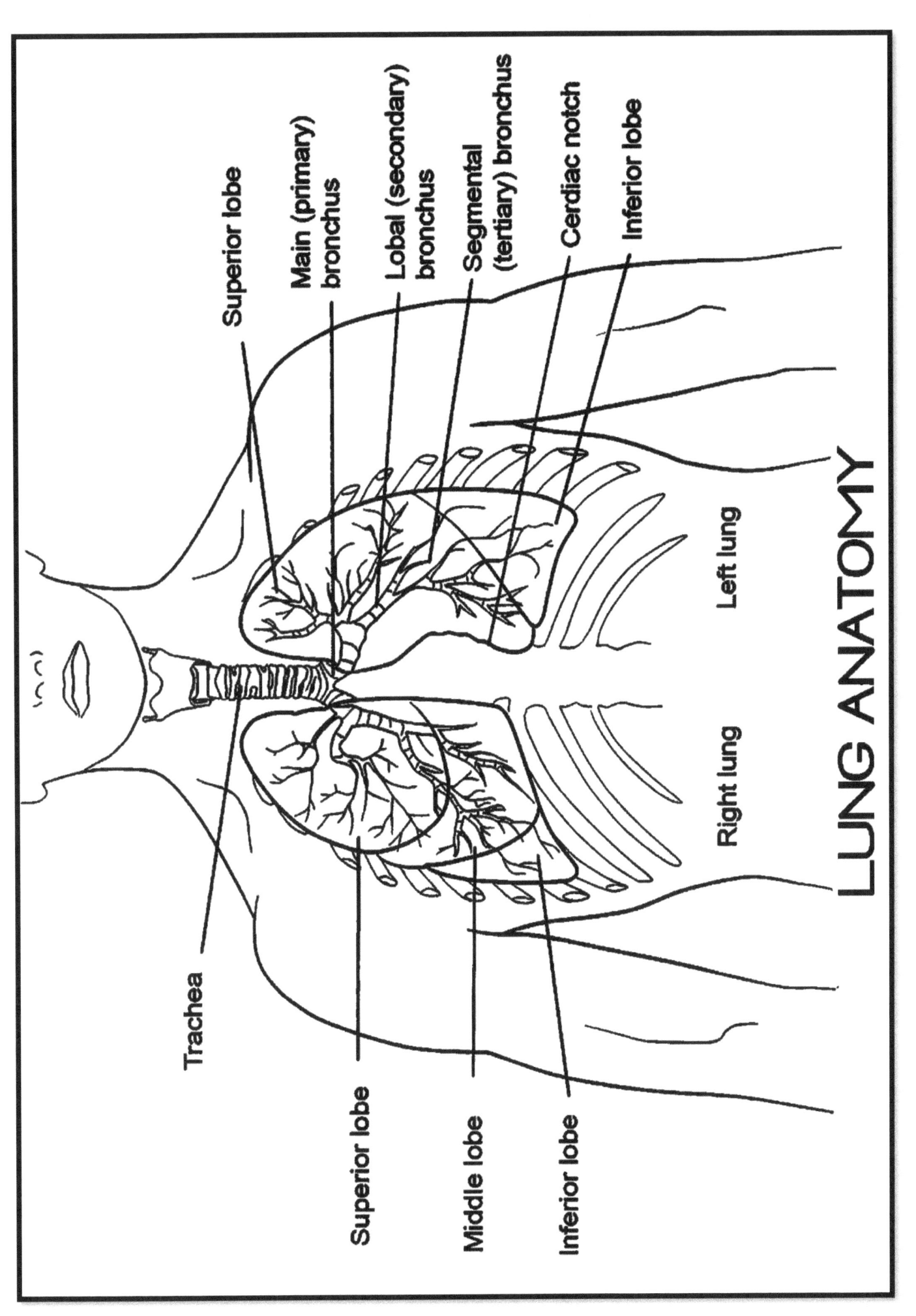

LUNG ANATOMY

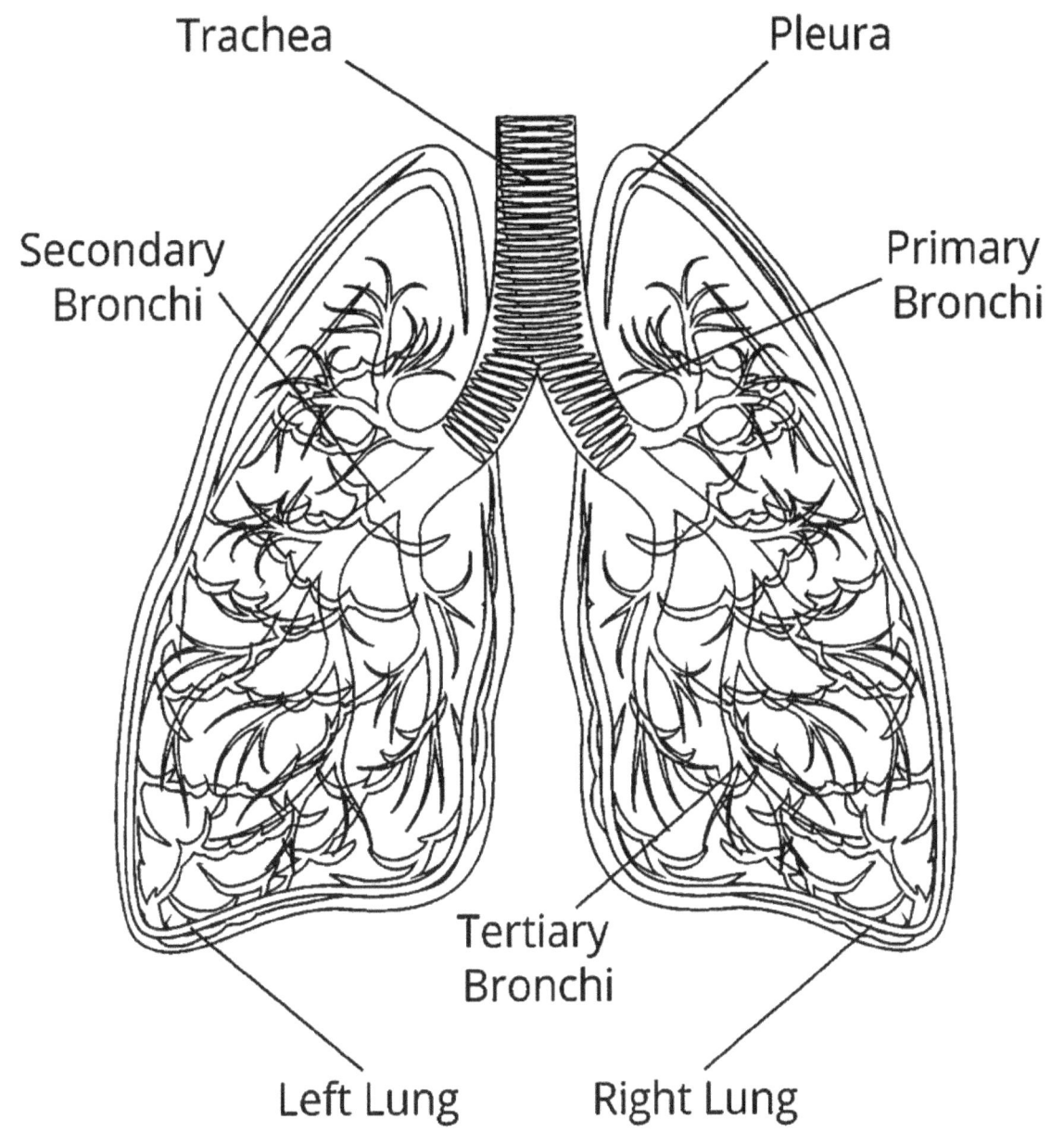

Trachea

Pleura

Secondary
Bronchi

Primary
Bronchi

Tertiary
Bronchi

Left Lung

Right Lung

LUNGS ANATOMY

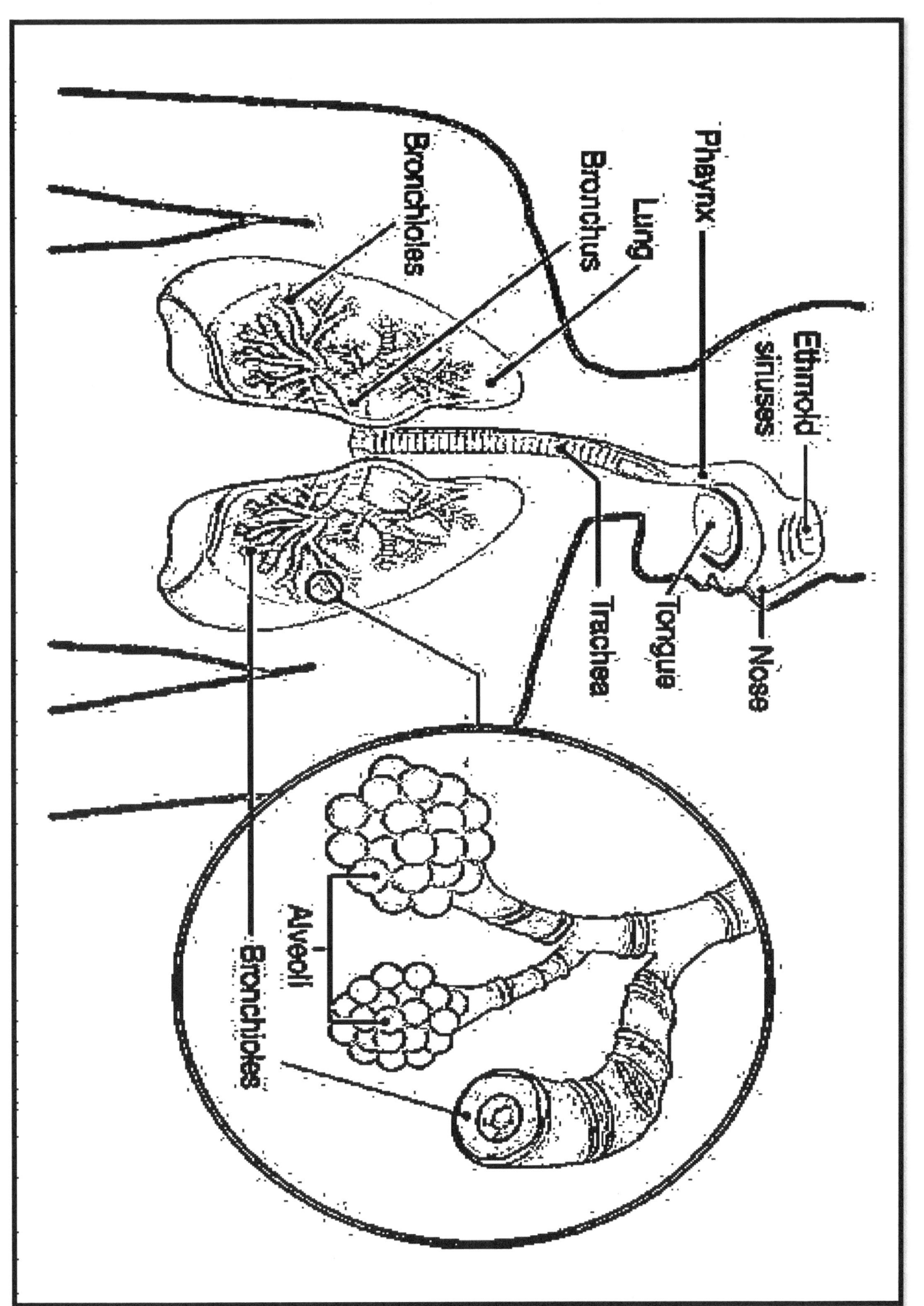

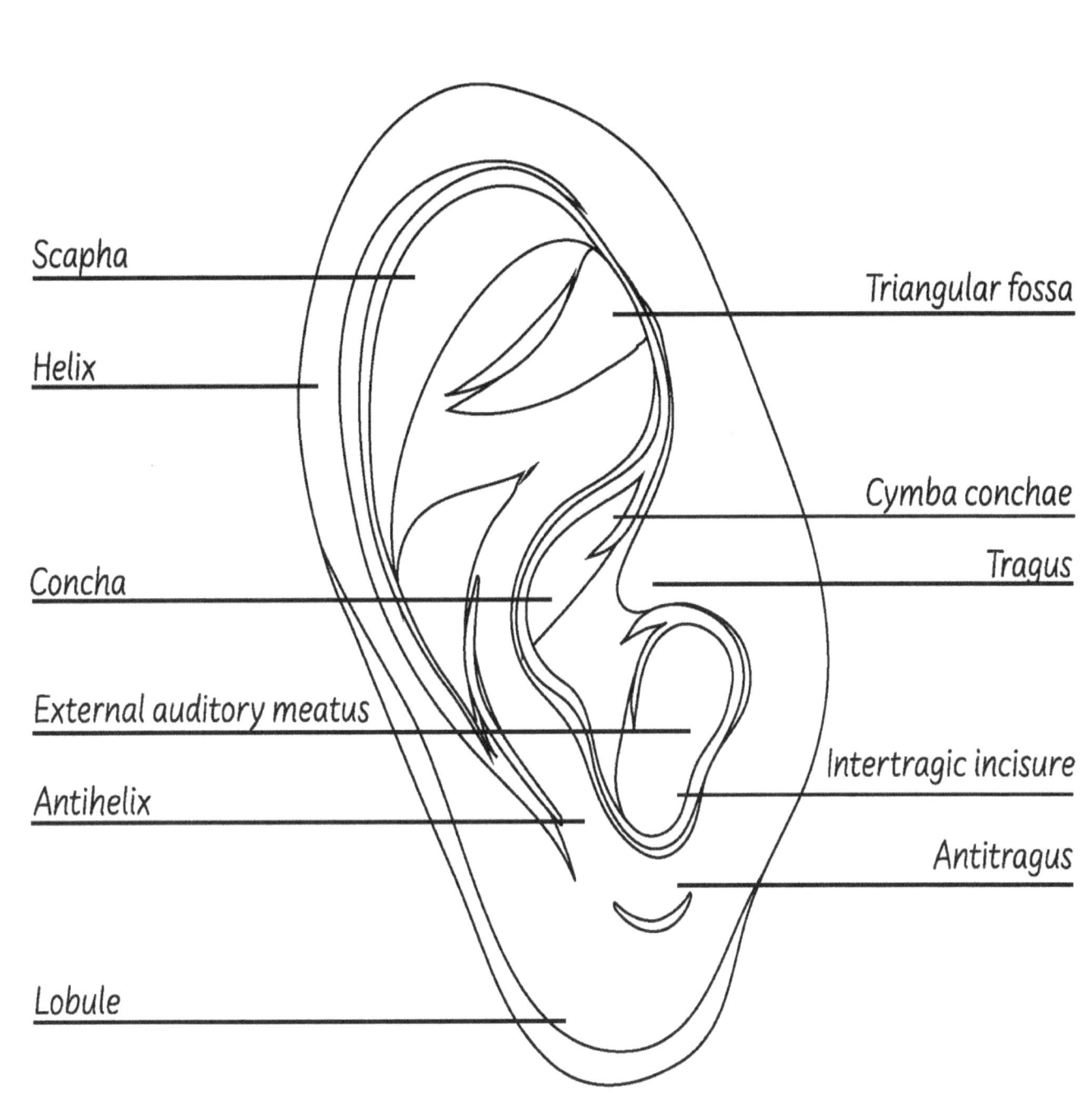

Scapha

Helix

Concha

External auditory meatus

Antihelix

Lobule

Triangular fossa

Cymba conchae

Tragus

Intertragic incisure

Antitragus

EAR ANATOMY

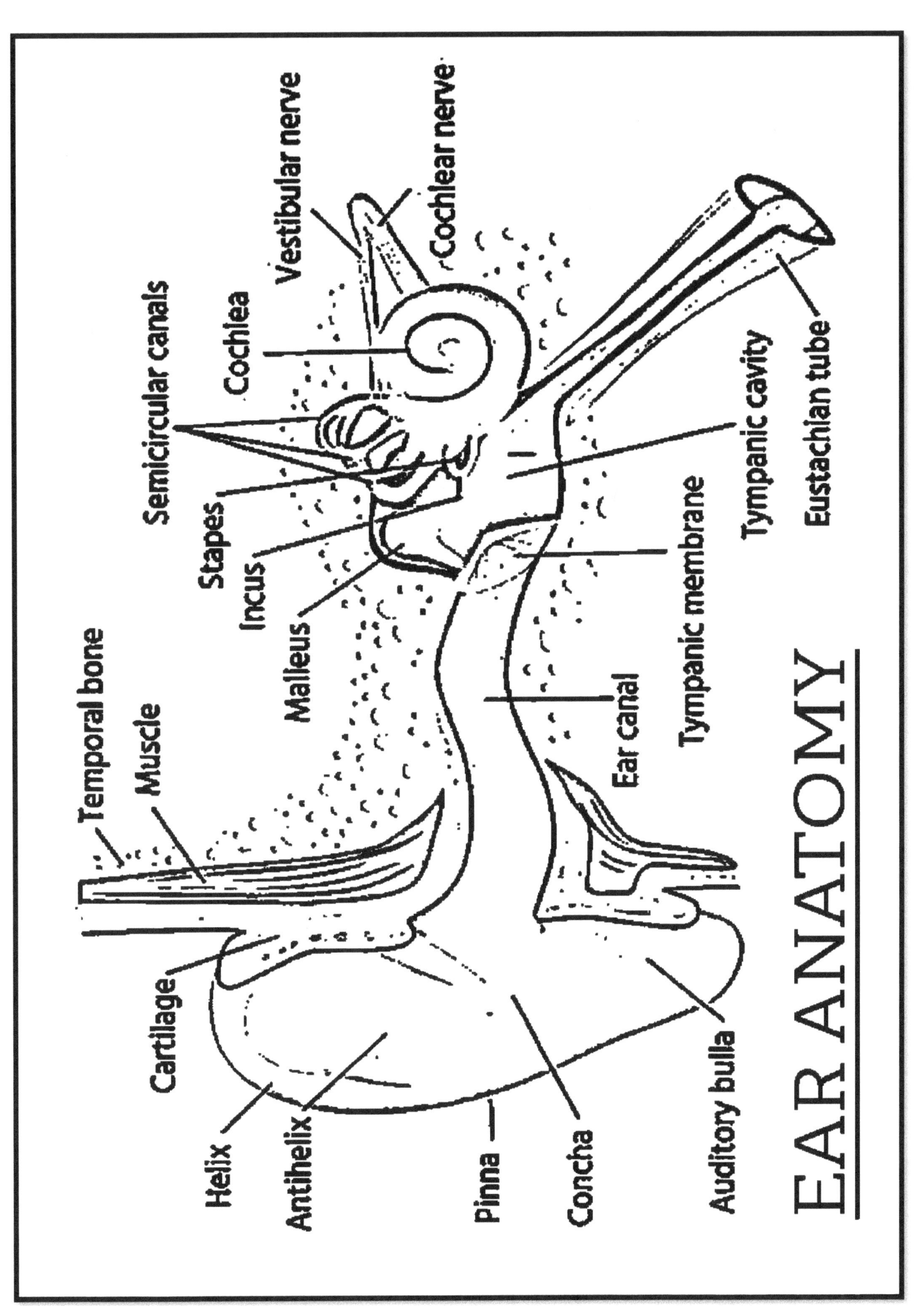

EAR ANATOMY

Vestibular nerve

Cochlear nerve

Semicircular canals

Cochlea

Stapes

Incus

Malleus

Temporal bone

Muscle

Tympanic cavity

Eustachian tube

Tympanic membrane

Ear canal

Cartilage

Helix

Antihelix

Pinna

Concha

Auditory bulla

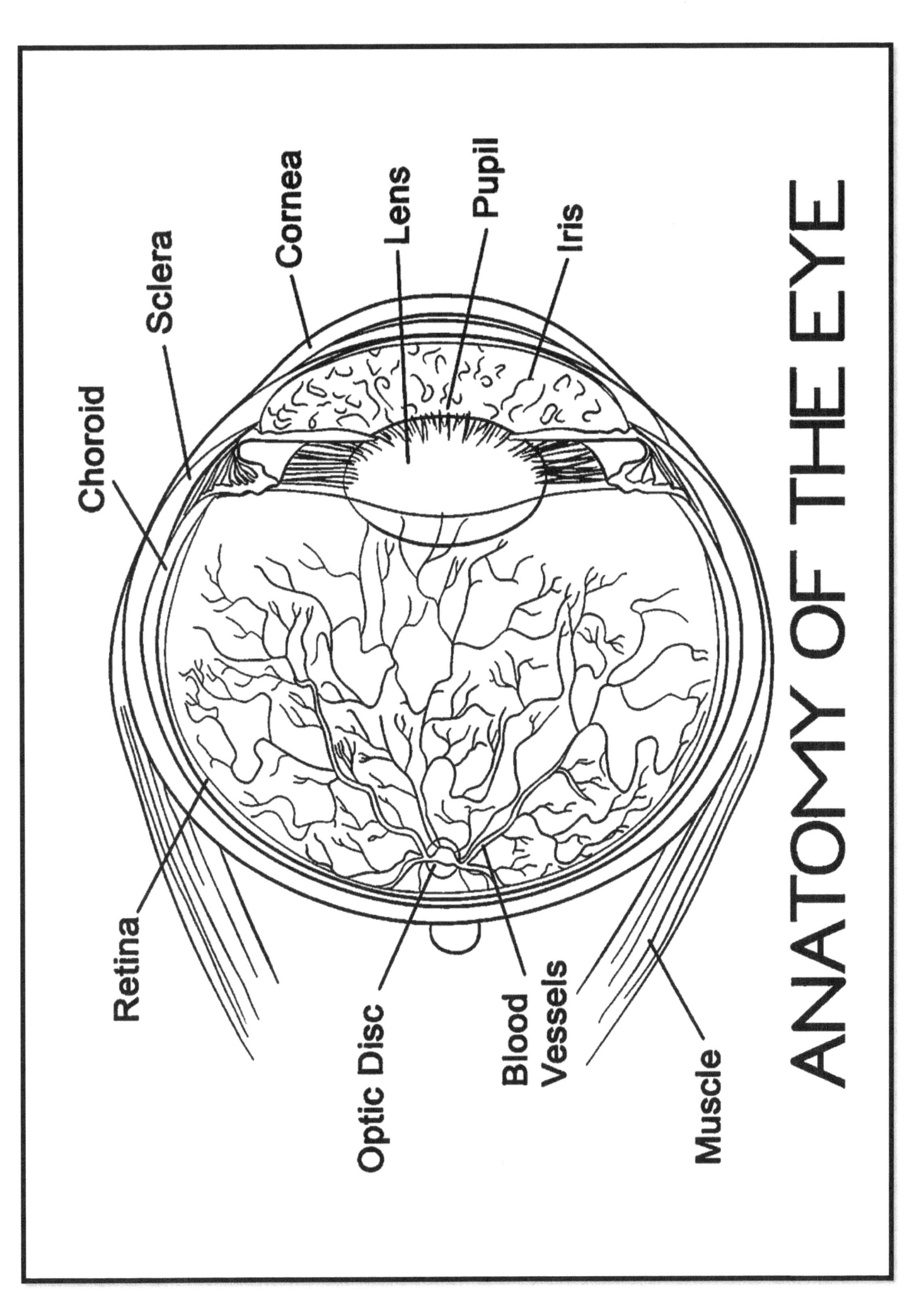

Choroid
Sclera
Cornea
Lens
Pupil
Iris
Retina
Optic Disc
Blood Vessels
Muscle

ANATOMY OF THE EYE

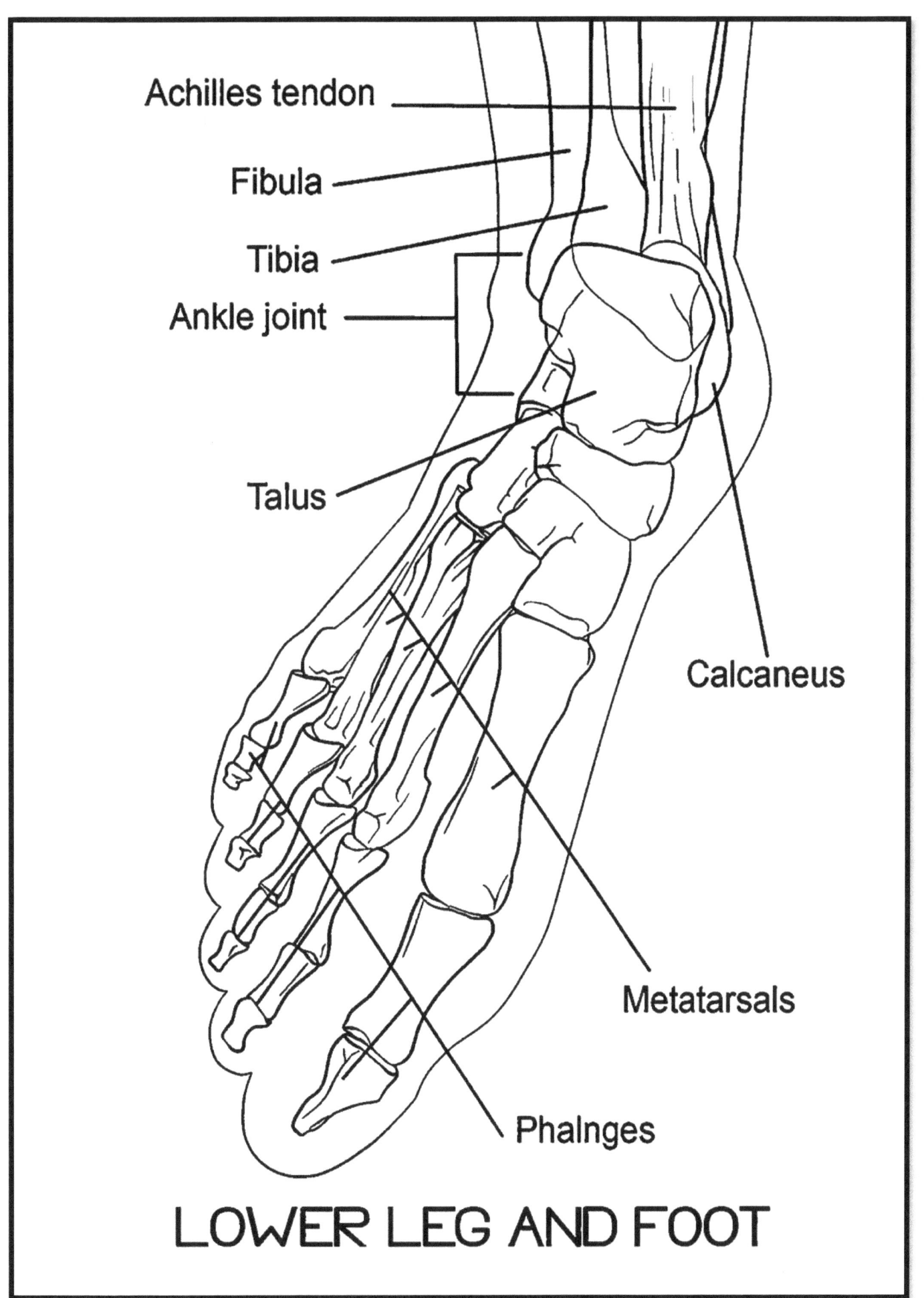

Achilles tendon

Fibula

Tibia

Ankle joint

Talus

Calcaneus

Metatarsals

Phalnges

LOWER LEG AND FOOT

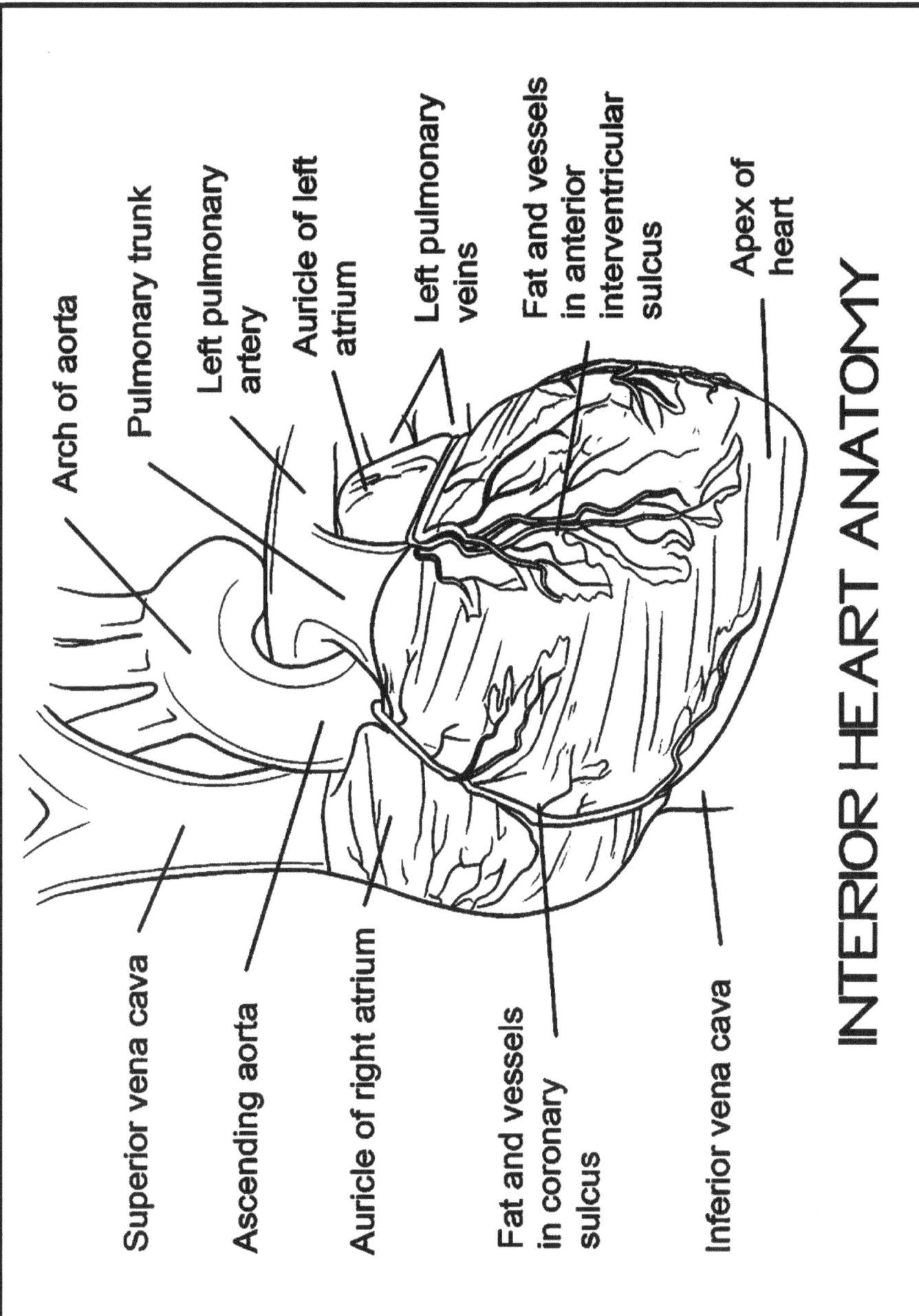

Arch of aorta

Pulmonary trunk

Left pulmonary artery

Auricle of left atrium

Left pulmonary veins

Fat and vessels in anterior interventricular sulcus

Apex of heart

Superior vena cava

Ascending aorta

Auricle of right atrium

Fat and vessels in coronary sulcus

Inferior vena cava

INTERIOR HEART ANATOMY

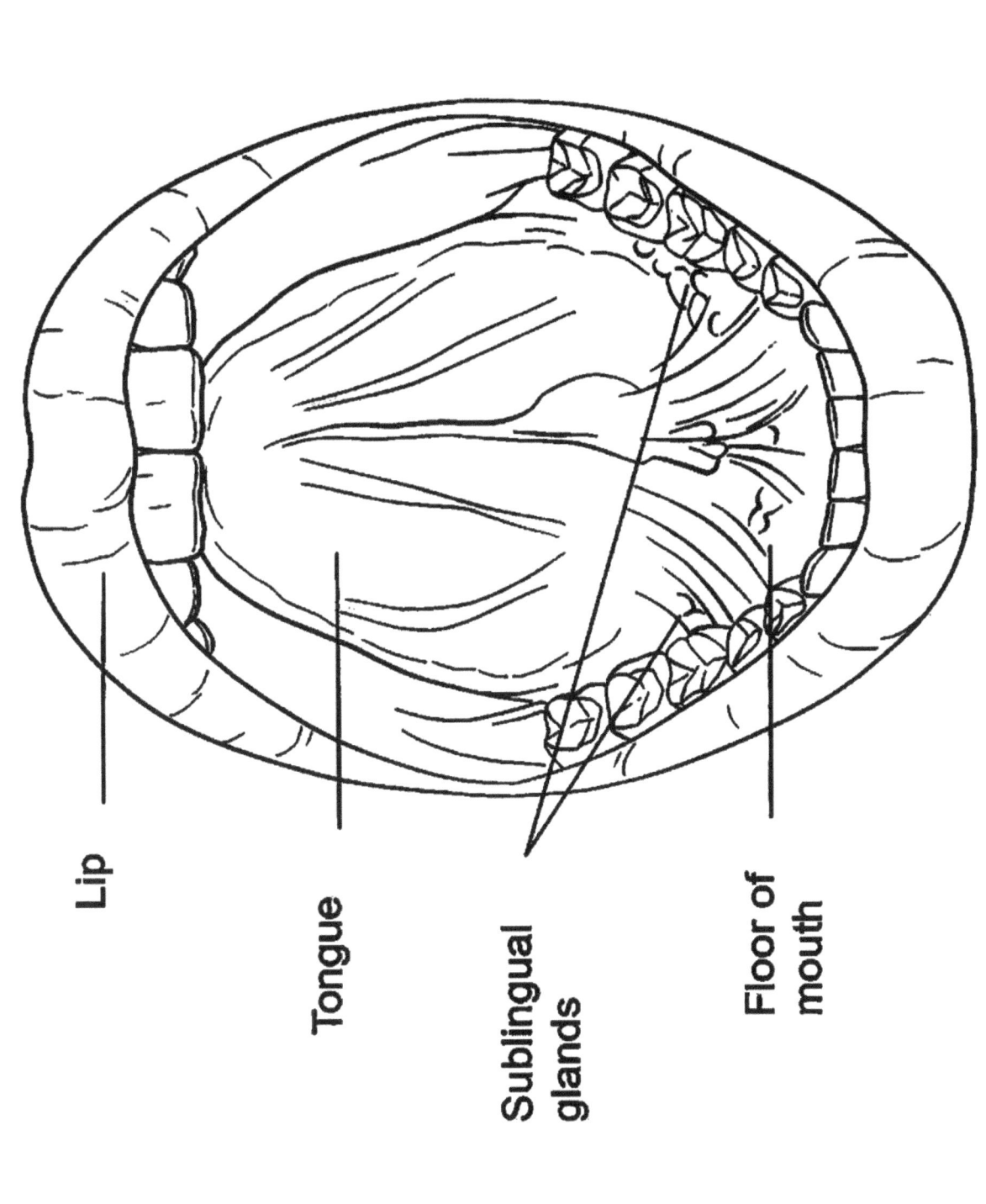

Lip

Tongue

Sublingual glands

Floor of mouth

MOUNTH AND TONGUE ANATOMY

KEDNEY ANATOMY

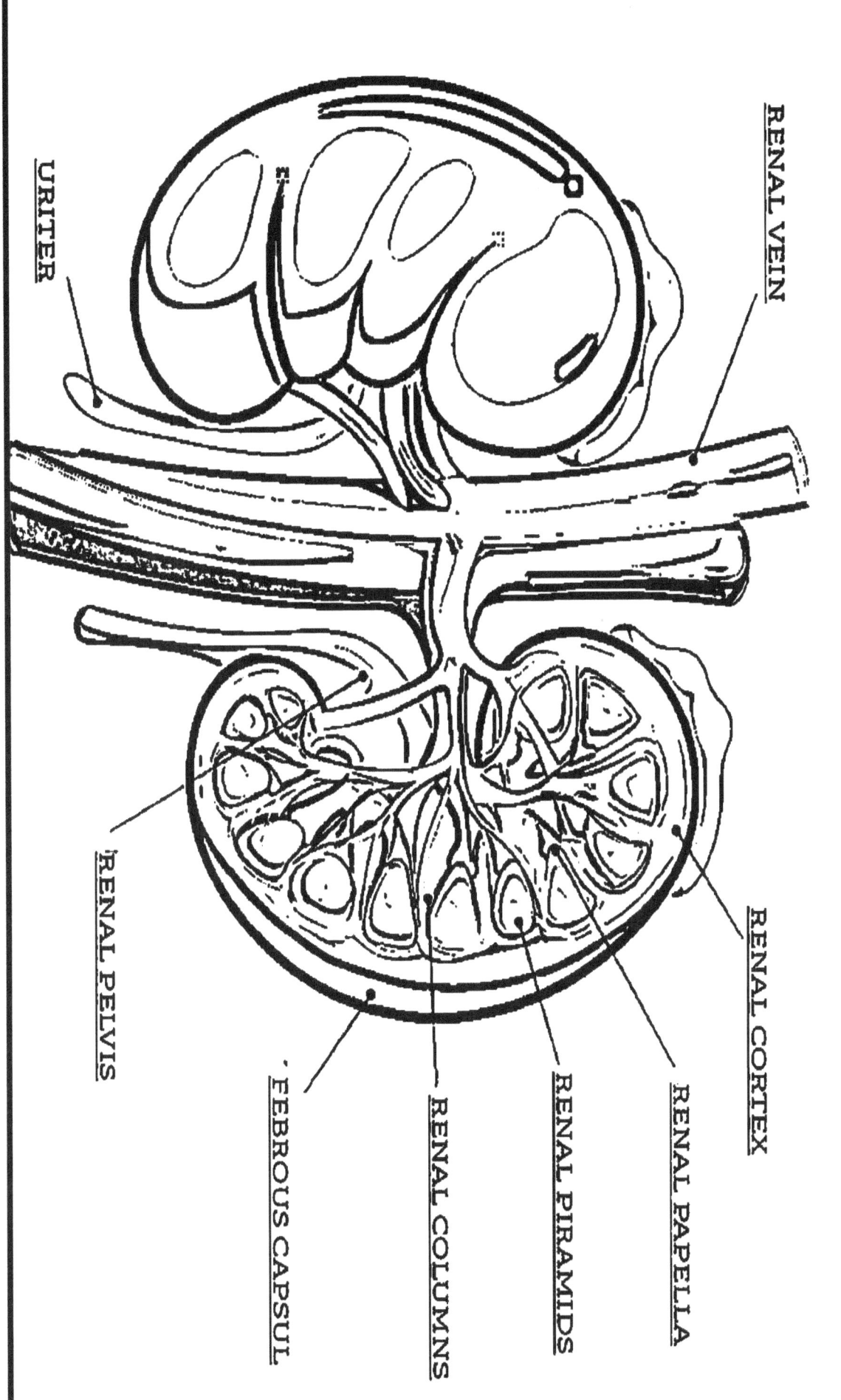

RENAL VEIN

URITER

RENAL PELVIS

RENAL CORTEX

FEBROUS CAPSUL

RENAL COLUMNS

RENAL PIRAMIDS

RENAL PAPELLA

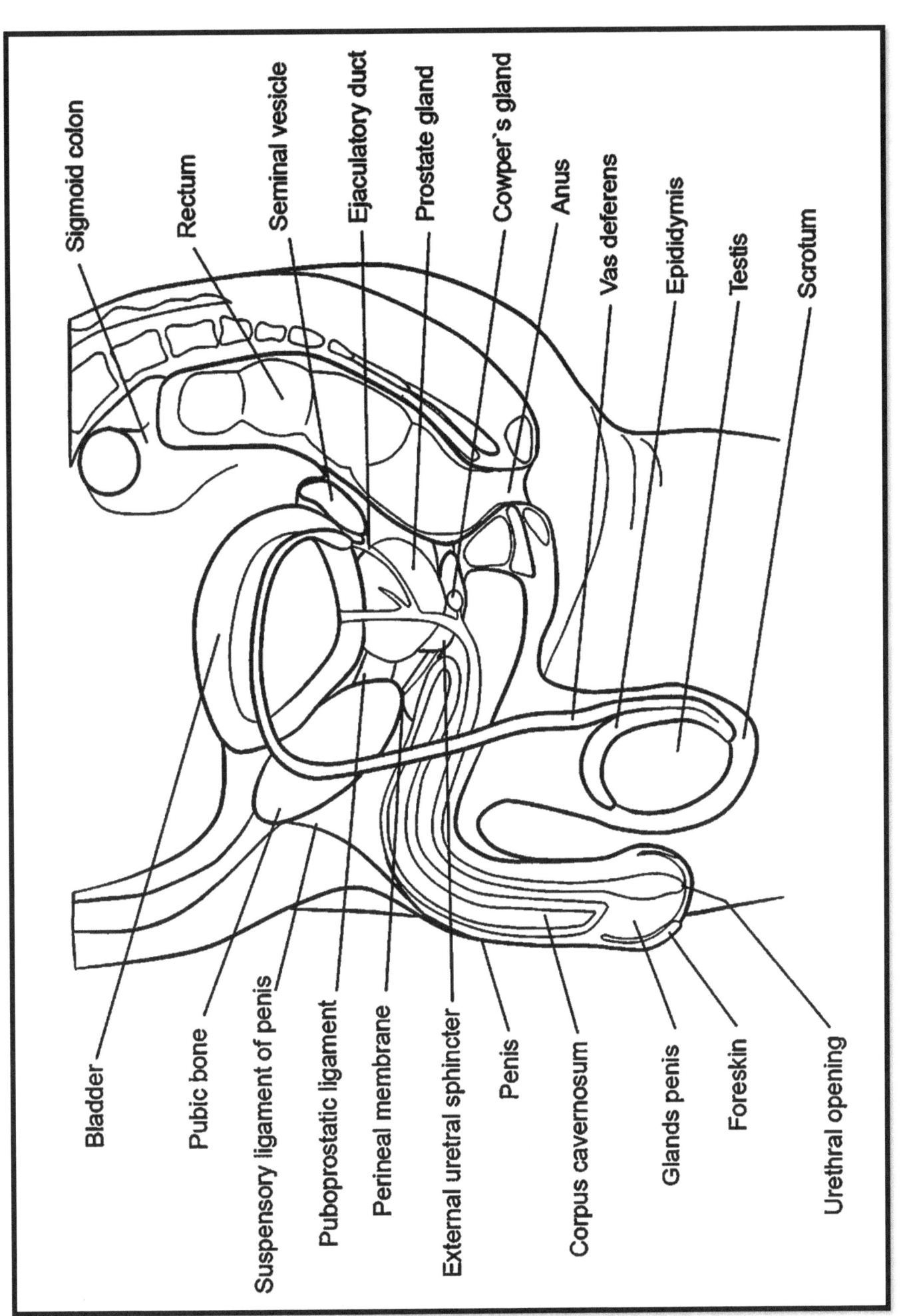

SHOULDER JOINT ANATOMY

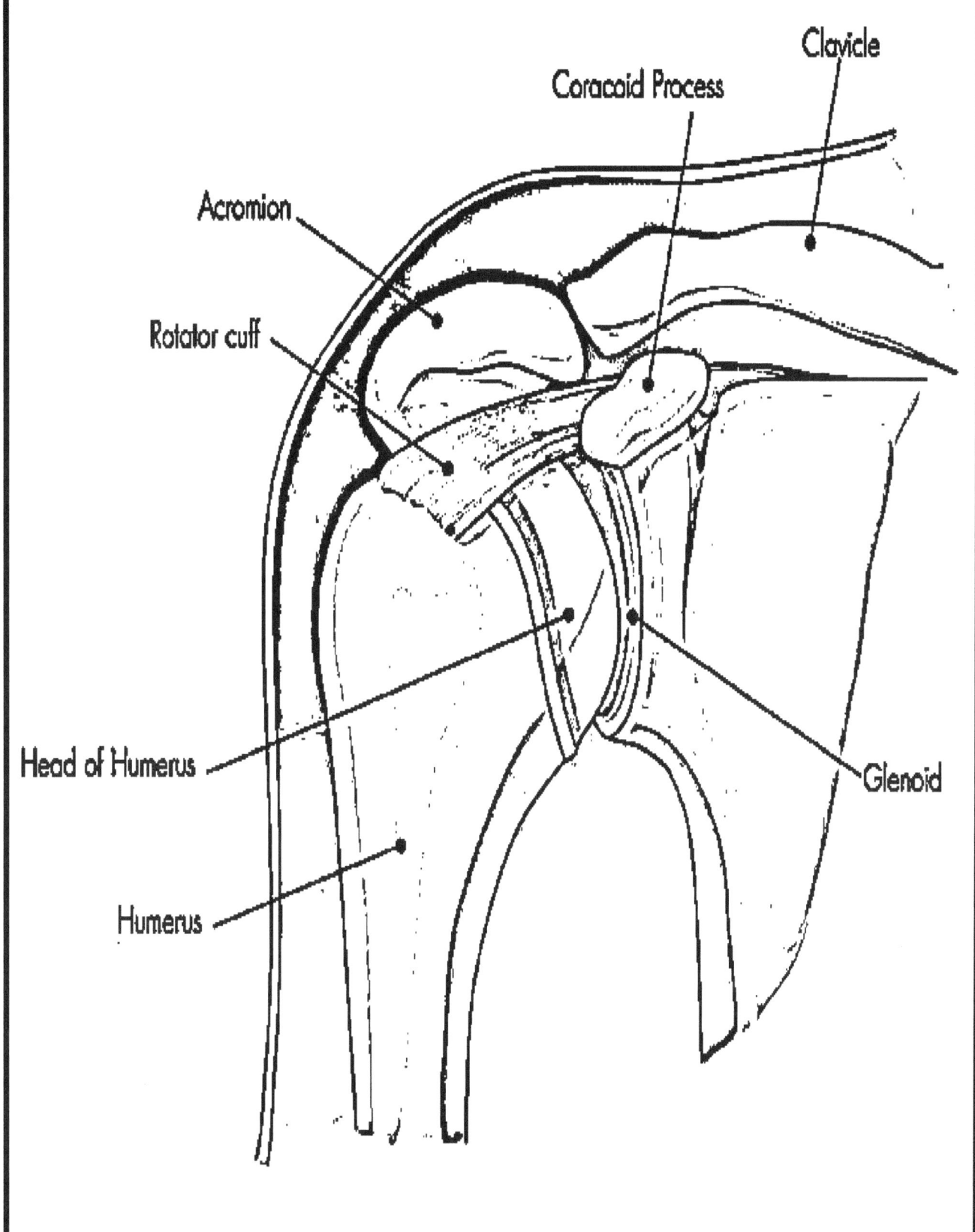

Clavicle

Coracoid Process

Acromion

Rotator cuff

Head of Humerus

Glenoid

Humerus